The
Immortality
Edge

Realize the Secrets of Your Telomeres for a Longer, Healthier Life

Michael Fossel, MD, PhD
Greta Blackburn
Dave Woynarowski, MD

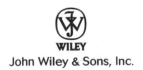

WILEY

John Wiley & Sons, Inc.

Published by John Wiley & Sons, Inc., Hoboken, New Jersey
Published simultaneously in Canada

Design by Forty-five Degree Design LLC

The information contained in this book is not intended to serve as a replacement for professional medical advice. Any use of the information in this book is at the reader's discretion. The author and the publisher specifically disclaim any and all liability arising directly or indirectly from the use or application of any information contained in this book. A health-care professional should be consulted regarding your specific situation.

For general information about our other products and services, please contact our Customer Care Department within the United States at (800) 762-2974, outside the United States at (317) 572-3993 or fax (317) 572-4002.

Wiley also publishes its books in a variety of electronic formats. Some content that appears in print may not be available in electronic books. For more information about Wiley products, visit our web site at www.wiley.com.

Library of Congress Cataloging-in-Publication Data:

Fossel, Michael.
    The immortality edge : realize the secrets of your telomeres for a longer, healthier life / Michael Fossel.
        p.   cm.
    Includes bibliographical references and index.
    ISBN 978-0-470-87390-8 (cloth); 978-0-470-92891-2 (ebk); 978-0-470-92892-9 (ebk); 978-0-470-92893-6 (ebk)
        1. Longevity—Popular works.   2. Longevity—Genetic aspects—Popular works.   3. Telomere—Popular works.   I. Title.
    RA776.75.F673 2010
    612.6'8—dc22

                                                            2010033498

Printed in the United States of America

10 9 8 7 6 5 4 3 2 1

To my mom, Sarah Blackburn: I wish we knew then what we know now. I will love you and miss you and your unconditional love forever, Gorgeous.

—Greta Blackburn

To all of our loved ones we didn't save, and to all of those we hope to save.

—Dave Woynarowski, MD

Here's to turning life on its head: sad nursing homes to glad chromosomes.

—Michael Fossel, MD, PhD

CONTENTS

PREFACE
by Dave Woynarowski, MD

In 1969, as astronaut Neil Armstrong took man's first steps on the moon, he famously said, "That's one small step for man, one giant leap for mankind." No words could be closer to describing the feeling I have about telomere biology and its huge impact on health and longevity.

The parallels to the space and lunar programs are many. The lunar landing gave rise to technology that we are still exploring and benefiting from today. In many ways it revolutionized our thinking and changed how we move about through the world. So it is with telomere biology.

Telomere biology is the first bastion of true longevity research. It encompasses all the prior theories on aging and drills down to the sub-molecular level to look at our genetic material and what happens to us because of who we are and what we do. Indeed, telomere biology is an extension of all of the other theories on aging—including wear and tear, antioxidant deficiency, genetic and hormonal deterioration, and mitochondrial aging and dysfunction—since ultimately they all point to the telomere.

If we are to believe what is coming out of the labs, telomere research will greatly enhance our potential health span and life-span, allowing us to continue our pursuits of life, liberty, and happiness far longer than even our most immediate ancestors did. If there ever was a missing link to health and longevity, telomere biology is it, and it's here right now staring us in the face—even daring us to use it.

Telomere research won the 2009 Nobel Prize and it has changed our understanding of longevity in ways that are meaningful to every man and woman—this is not just esoteric disease research that will take years to bear fruit. Even more refreshing is the way that telomere research has embraced the way we live our lives every day. By ramping up our cells' health and longevity we can prevent disease and aging rather than relying on pharmaceutical science to fix us when we wear out and break.

This book shows how we can do many simple, meaningful, practical things that do not involve costly or dangerous drugs, things that can yield almost immediate benefits in how we look, feel, and move through the world. We can do these things ourselves! Consider these facts:

- There is solid and seductively simple and repeatable science to justify the use of supplements both to prolong telomere length and to lengthen the shortest, most critical telomeres.
- Solid research validates the effects of meditation and stress reduction on cell biology and telomere length.
- Irrefutable evidence links most of the disease of aging directly and/or indirectly to telomere length.
- The effects of exercise in telomere length are also well documented.

This gives us everyday tools that all of us can apply to make a real impact on our health and most likely our longevity as well.

Telomere biology represents a paradigm shift in medical and health research as it allows the power of science to be directly harnessed by everyday people, removing it from the ivory tower bastions of scientific debate and rhetoric. Applying that power to your everyday life is our primary goal in presenting to you *The Immortality Edge*.

I know in my heart that *The Immortality Edge* is at the very least a small step, the first of many bigger and faster steps that will lead us to what people have dreamed of since they were able to ponder their own mortality: a long and truly healthy life.

PREFACE
by Michael Fossel, MD, PhD

Many scientists (Nobel Prizes notwithstanding) have been quick to argue that the telomere—nongenetic material that determines the life span of a cell—isn't important because telomeres don't cause aging. This is an argument that few (including me) would disagree with, but it's an argument that wildly misses the point. Causation isn't the issue.

Telomeres don't cause aging—they really don't—yet they play a central role in timing and in controlling the aging process. Armchair philosophers want to argue causes; the rest of us want cures. When my home is in flames, I don't want a debate about the cause of the fire; I want to save my house.

Because I am a physician, my interest in aging is not academic but purely practical. Talking about the cause of aging may be interesting. It might even be useful, but interest and usefulness can be measured only by what you can do about it. If you can't actually change something, why talk about it?

In real life, medicine is not philosophy; it is an exploration of what works, what's practical. I don't want causes—I want interventions! When people are sick, they do not come to me looking only for a diagnosis; they come for treatment. If making a diagnosis contributes to finding a treatment, then it is useful. If an explanation helps to maintain my health, it is useful. But the cause, the diagnosis, the explanation, the philosophy, or the academic knowledge has little intrinsic use, except as it improves our personal lives. Discussions about the causes of aging are fun, but interventions are much more useful to anyone who is aging—which, incidentally, includes you and me.

So can we use telomeres to reverse aging? Reversing aging requires an effective intervention. Claims about reversing aging, like other fairy tales, have been around since humans first began to talk to one another, and these claims are found in our earliest recorded stories, including *The Epic of Gilgamesh*, written almost five thousand years ago.

Given the record to date, it is not surprising that the possibility of reversing aging inspires eternal optimism, always quickly dashed by an equally eternal pessimism that is based on inconvenient facts. Reality always, sooner or later, trumps wishful thinking. Until now, fairy tales about reversing aging have always been nothing more than fairy tales.

Once, while giving a talk at the National Institutes of Health, I said, "Anyone who leaves here thinking we can reverse human aging is an idiot; anyone who leaves here thinking we can't reverse human aging is an idiot. If you're reasonable, you'll be uncertain when you walk out the door." We should be uncertain. If I live to be two hundred years old and I'm still healthy, I'll be thrilled but still uncertain. The false claims have too long a human history. Maybe I'll live only another fifty years!

But here's what we do know: we can already reverse aging in human cells, and we can already reverse aging in simple human tissues. What we don't know for sure is whether we can reverse aging in *you*. However, given what we now know about the role of telomeres and telomerase, the enzyme that makes telomeres grow, shorn of preconceptions and debates about causes, the answer is yes, we probably can.

If we reset telomere lengths in cells or in tissues, we can reverse aging in those cells and tissues. Currently, we are just about able to reset telomere lengths in your body. We have several compounds that promise exactly that, and we are rapidly finding more (and more effective) compounds.

If we could go forward a century and ask an average person when people first "cured" human aging, the date will be somewhere in the current decade; not fifty years from now, but now. People in the near future will remember the first effective treatment for human aging—the earliest users of TA-65 and of the other compounds now still in the labs—that allowed us to enjoy long healthy lives, active lives, without Alzheimer's, heart attacks, strokes, arthritis, dependence, or nursing homes.

Health is not simply avoiding the consequences of aging, and avoiding aging is certainly not simply about taking a pill. Our doctors and our grandmothers have been giving us advice for years on how to stay healthy—not that we pay much attention. All of us know that diet, exercise, and avoiding stress go a long way toward improving our lives. In this book, we're going to explore all of these and a lot more, paying particular attention to those things that have been proven to reduce the pace of telomere shortening. Before we do, however, let me give you two pieces of practical advice.

The first is that we don't all agree on what is best, and that is actually reasonable and probably healthy. You may have noticed that advice changes over time, and humility is probably a useful thing. Just prior to 1900, many medical scientists were advocating sugar as "nature's perfect food," a suggestion we find amusing and probably dangerous. It's likely that you and I will, if we live another century, look back on much of what we currently "know" to be healthy and wonder how we could have been so credulous and silly.

The second piece of advice is related to the first: moderation in all things, even moderation. If you're sure that something is good for you, don't take it too seriously, or your seriousness alone might kill you.

Go easy on trying to stay healthy, or you won't succeed. Every year or two I see a patient who comes in complaining of dangerously high blood pressure. "My blood pressure is so high that I'm afraid I'll have a stroke! Quick, you've got to *do* something!" I ask this person how he knows his blood pressure is so high. "Because I've been taking my blood pressure every ten minutes all day at home. And now it's getting *higher*!" My advice? Stop taking your blood pressure so often.

Chill out, ignore your fear, and go watch the moon rise. If you really want to stay healthy, don't take it all so seriously. If the only way you can guarantee a healthy life is by eating sawdust, forget it and have some chocolate mousse instead. Don't stay up at night worrying about how to fall asleep; don't exercise so hard you hurt yourself. People have never lived past one hundred by ignoring the life in their lives. So we'll give you advice, probably good advice, but don't let it prevent you from living your life.

ACKNOWLEDGMENTS

The three of us would like to acknowledge David Bunnell who, working against short deadlines, helped us write and organize the material in this book and worked tirelessly as we moved toward a final manuscript. A pioneer of the personal computer industry, David has transformed himself into an avid member of the life extension revolution.

—Michael Fossel, MD, PhD; Greta Blackburn; David Woynarowski, MD

My thanks to Greta for making us do this, to Dave W. for going along with it, to David B. for actually doing it, and to all those current readers who will still be around with us two hundred years from now. And to chocolate, of course, the true secret of immortality.

—Michael Fossel, MD, PhD

Thanks to Dr. Edmund Chein for hosting a conference in Palm Springs more than ten years ago. Thanks also to Dr. Jerry T. Shay for his brilliant presentation at that event, during which he discussed the Geron Corporation's telomere technology and studies. It was not long after that a friend, Noel Thomas Patton, whom I had invited to the event, got involved with Geron and eventually obtained a license for their telomerase activator, TA-65. Out of my efforts in helping to get TA Sciences off the ground, I had the good luck to meet the key players responsible for the foundational principles in this book.

Michael Fossel, MD, PhD, wrote *Reversing Human Aging* in 1997. When I asked him, somewhat timidly, if he was interested in working with me on a book about telomeres and their significance to aging he almost immediately responded in the affirmative. Dr. David Woynarowski was an attendee at an age-management conference when we met. He was an ultra-runner who was about to turn fifty himself, and his enthusiasm about telomere biology had grown since he first read about it in research papers. I knew that he had the ability to generate copy that translated esoteric science into easy-to-understand concepts. The final product is only as good as each member of its team. My team was exceptional. Thanks, guys.

The final challenge facing us was how to blend three voices with three different sets of experience and knowledge. Plus there was heavy lifting needed to collate all of the science and all of the information and make it cohesive. David Bunnell is our heavy lifter. Without his talent, experience, knowledge, and work ethic this book would not exist. We all owe him a huge thank you and could not possibly have gotten this book done and on deadline without him.

There are many contributors to this book without whom *The Immortality Edge* would not exist, including Coleen O'Shea, our agent, and Tom Miller, our editor at John Wiley & Sons. Thanks for believing in us and in telomere biology! Very special thanks to production editor Lisa Burstiner at Wiley for her support, patience, and expertise at copy editing. During the final weeks of getting the book ready to go to press things might have fallen through the cracks without her guidance. Thanks also to copy editor Judith Antonelli.

Thank you to all of the pioneers in the field, without whom our book would have no foundation in science. Thank you,

Dr. Calvin Harley, formerly of Geron Corporation, for your understanding of the relationship between telomeres and the Hayflick Limit. Without that understanding none of many of the discoveries in telomere biology would have practical applications. Bill Andrews, PhD, thanks not only for your codiscovery of the hTert gene, but for your friendship, energy, and support over the years. Your unflagging pursuit of the cure to aging is an inspiration and benefit to all of us. Plus, you are one heck of an ultra-runner. And thanks to your dad, Ralph Andrews, the eighty-something television pioneer, activist, and author who still exercises daily and looks decades younger than his years and who motivated you to go out into the world and work to fight the aging process.

Thanks to those who continually push the envelope and work tirelessly for this cause: Aubrey de Grey, PhD; Michael West, PhD; and our great friend David Kekich, founder of the Maximum Life Foundation. Big thanks to the Life Extension Foundation for paving the way with supplements and information that have helped us all stay healthy for decades. In particular, thanks to William Faloon, cofounder of LEF, for his unflagging enthusiasm and support for all things eternal.

Family members and friends of all the authors were key to sustaining the writing and creative effort. Cathy Woynarowski held down the fort for her brother Dr. Dave as he spent hours working on this project. Joy Fossel, wife of Michael and a meticulous lawyer, was a tremendous resource as contracts and legal matters arose. My adorable poodle puppy, Romeo, spent many a lonesome hour staring at me plaintively yet patiently. Without the forever support of my BFF Laura Neftin there were many times when I might have lost steam. Also, my great buddy Michael "the Rock" Crecco was there to assist with whatever administrative chores needed doing when deadlines loomed, personalities flared and clashed, and energy dwindled. We could not have made this happen without your ongoing support.

Thanks to my Dad, Bill Blackburn, for handing down some cool genes and for being among the first to supplement with

TA-65. At age eighty-nine he is still going strong, golfing, and spending time with his fantastic wife, Shirley. I won't ever forget when, six months into his telomerase activation program, he told me, "I feel great! I have more energy and I can even bend over and pick up my golf balls more easily. I suppose you're going to say it's those vitamins you have me taking."

—Greta Blackburn

Thanks to William Andrews, PhD, for starting me on my telomere journey and helping me understand the steps—and for his huge contributions to the field of longevity that have gone largely unheralded until now.

To coauthor Greta Blackburn for your incredible ideas, insights, and fortitude as well as your connections to all the right people, which allowed me to be where I am at this moment.

To coauthor Michael Fossel, MD, PhD, for keeping it all in perspective.

To Tom Miller at John Wiley & Sons for raising your hand and understanding the huge importance of this work!

To David Bunnell for your writing and organizational excellence.

—David Woynarowski, MD

The Hunt for Immortality

Telomere [TEL-uh-meer, TEE-luh-meer] (noun): the segment of DNA that occurs at the ends of chromosomes.

Telomerase [tuh-LO-muh-reys] (noun): an enzyme that
causes telomeres to lengthen; facilitates cell division and
may account for the immortality of some cells.

On the morning of October 5, 2009, Carol Greider was at home
doing her laundry, thinking about the Spin class she was going to
take later on with two female friends. She was tired from long
hours at her lab on the campus of the Johns Hopkins School of
Medicine and was happy to have a day off. It was a relief to let her
mind relax from all the research work and the intense pressure of
being one of the country's foremost female scientists.

Then Greider got a very unexpected phone call—the kind of
phone call that most professors, most peace activists, and even
some world leaders dream about but rarely receive.

After the call, Greider's mind was racing a million miles a second; she wasn't sure what to do. Soon, she figured, she might
be getting a few more calls from media organizations and from

friends and colleagues. So the first thing she did was send an e-mail to her fitness-class friends: "I'm sorry I can't Spin right now. I've won the Nobel Prize."

Greider's Nobel Prize in medicine was to be shared with her former professor at the University of California–Berkeley, Elizabeth Blackburn, and with Harvard geneticist Jack Szostak. It was awarded to them for the pioneering research they did in the role of telomeres and chromosomes and for the discovery Greider and Blackburn made back in 1984 of telomerase, an enzyme that causes the ends of chromosomes to grow. In reporting on the Nobel Prize, the *New York Times* said that the existence of telomerase has a "deep relevance" for both cancer and aging. In the opinion of the authors of this book, this is, in fact, an understatement. What these remarkable scientists discovered will inevitably lead to a universal cure for all forms of cancer, but even more than this, they have indeed discovered the very secret of immortality.

Contrary to the conventional myth that the only proven ways to extend life expectancy are through severe restrictive practices—such as the calorie-reduction diet—that most can't and don't want to follow, there is now a far better, more effective way. Thanks to recent profound breakthroughs in DNA research that go well beyond the initial discoveries that led to the Nobel Prize, it is now possible for you to extend your life expectancy beyond 100 years to 120 or more (perhaps even indefinitely) while leading an active, robust, independent lifestyle, maintaining all the strength and vitality you had when you were much younger. Imagine being a centenarian looking half your age, playing outdoors with your great-grandchildren, dancing with much younger partners, enjoying new hobbies and pursuits, and, yes, still having a great sex life—all without having to worry about life-threatening conditions like cancer, heart disease, diabetes, chronic infections, dementia, poor eyesight, hearing loss, low energy, and the other miserable conditions that plague too many older people. It may sound too good to be true, but it isn't.

Until now, the concept of immortality was considered forever unachievable. Over time, the cells in our bodies reach a stage at which they can no longer reproduce themselves—a retirement-like state in which they die or no longer divide and thus become inert. This end point is called *senescence*. The effect of senescent cells appears very obviously when they accumulate in quite large numbers in just one tissue (the cartilage in our joints), but even in small numbers they pose a disproportionate, although less obvious, threat to the surrounding healthy tissues because of their steadily deteriorating metabolic state.

Senescent cells secrete abnormally large amounts of certain proteins that are harmful to their neighbors, stimulating excessive growth and degrading normal tissue architecture. These changes appear to promote the progression of age-related diseases, including cancer. (Although cancer sometimes strikes younger people and even children, the overwhelming number of cancer cases occur in the elderly.) Senescent cells in our skin make us look withered. In our immune system, they make us susceptible to the diseases of aging such as heart disease, heart failure, diabetes, and fragility. Even if we are lucky enough to avoid these calamities, eventually so many of our cells will be in a state of senescence that the body as a whole will no longer be able to sustain itself. When this happens, we die of "old age."

"Death is inevitable!" How many times have you heard this statement?

No matter how well you take care of yourself, what you eat, how great your genes are, or how lucky you are, it is impossible, scientists have thought, for any human being to live past 120. (This is called the Hayflick limit.) Indeed, the oldest man, as far as we have been able to verify without dispute, Christian Mortensen, lived to be 115, and the oldest woman, Jeanne Calment, barely squeaked past the theoretical Hayflick limit by reaching age 122 before passing away in 1997.

At that time, Leonard Hayflick, a professor of microbiology at Stanford University, and other scientists didn't know exactly why human cells divided only a limited number of times; perhaps it had to do with free radicals, the accumulation of mutations, a genetic switch that is flipped to the off position after we are too old to reproduce, changes in hormone regulation, the decreased efficiency of the immune system, or even divine providence. No one knew for sure.

Fast-forward to today, and thanks to our Nobel Prize winners and others, we now know exactly why living cells, except cancer cells and germ cells, become senescent, and even more exciting, we know how to increase the number of times cells can divide. In fact, we know how to make normal cells, as opposed to cancer cells, divide and live forever—to indeed become immortal.

This bears repeating. Living cells, including human ones, never have to die, never have to reach senescence. Understanding why isn't that complicated; it has nothing to do with stem cells, the reversal of gene expression, or mitochondria.

As most high school students know (or should know), the nucleus of every single cell in our bodies includes forty-six long twisted strands of DNA on which genes are found. These strands—called *chromosomes*—are organized in pairs, one chromosome in each pair coming from our mother and one coming from our father. Under powerful electronic microscopes, chromosomes look something like very tiny double sausages.

The DNA contained in chromosomes defines everything about us, from our hair color to our gender to the length of our little fingers. Chromosomes are important to all forms of life—indeed, they are found in every living thing, every living cell.

Solving the End-Replication Problem

When cells divide and multiply, it is very important that the DNA in the chromosomes remains intact; otherwise, genetic defects can occur, some not so serious and others very serious—some even causing cells to become cancerous. For many years, James

Watson, who with his partner, Francis Crick, with contributions from Rosalind Franklin, discovered the double-helix structure of DNA, wondered how DNA is protected when chromosomes divide and multiply. If we lost portions of the information encoded in our DNA every time it replicated, human life would be impossible. Our cells couldn't divide enough times to even allow us to be born. Watson thought about this, because the method a chromosome uses to replicate itself during cell division should, logically, destroy some of the genes at the ends of the DNA. Watson called this the *end-replication problem*.

By the mid-1970s, scientists knew the answer to this puzzle. There was general agreement that both ends of every chromosome contain relatively long strands of "junk" DNA called *telomeres*. The primary function of these telomeres, which consist of up to fifteen thousand repeats (in embryo cells) of the DNA sequence TTAGGG, appeared to be to protect the functional DNA. Thus, when chromosomes divide and multiply, instead of losing the DNA that matters, they lose only some of the telomere's DNA. With every replication of our DNA, part of the telomere sequence is chopped off. This is how nature protects the DNA in a chromosome.

One way to describe telomeres is to compare them to aglets, the plastic caps at the ends of shoelaces. Just as aglets keep shoelaces from falling apart at the end, telomeres keep the ends of DNA from fraying.

Today we can measure the age of cells by the length of the telomeres. Infants have long telomeres, but not quite as long as those found in human embryos. When we are conceived, the embryo has about fifteen thousand base pairs in its telomeres. After many replications, a newborn human is formed and born with approximately ten thousand base pairs in each telomere sequence. Thus, in the uterine development of a human, when cells are dividing furiously to make a newborn baby, five thousand base pairs of telomere length are lost. In a sense, we start to die the minute we are conceived! Adults have shorter telomeres; adults who are destined to live a long time have longer telomeres than do adults who are destined to live not so long.

There is even a disease of short telomeres: Werner's syndrome, more commonly known as progeria. The unfortunate people who are born with this rare disease age prematurely and have an average life expectancy of only twenty years. Researchers at the University of California–Davis found that male carriers of the gene that causes progeria (Fragile X syndrome), when compared to men their own age, have shorter telomeres than those who aren't carriers.

"Since we adjusted for age, we know that the telomere length is telling us something more than chronological age," said Dr. Ramin Farzaneh-Far, a cardiologist at the University of California–San Francisco who analyzed the data. "Hopefully it is measuring biological age."

Researchers at the Albert Einstein College of Medicine of Yeshiva University in New York City made an even bigger breakthrough with a large study of homogeneous Ashkenazi Jews who had previously been genetically studied. Comparing healthy elders who averaged ninety-seven years of age with their children and with the children of Ashkenazi Jews who had died at age eighty or younger, the researchers discovered a link between longevity and the presence of longer telomeres. The children of the older group consistently had longer telomeres than the children of those who had died at age eighty or younger.

Shorter telomeres don't correlate only with age, they also correlate with the stage of one's health. Another study found that among 780 patients with stable heart disease, people with the shortest telomeres in their immune cells had twice the risk of death and heart failure after 4.4 years as did patients with the longest telomeres. Those in the highest-risk group had telomeres half the length of those in the lowest-risk group.

These are just a few of dozens of studies and research projects that correlate telomere length to disease and to death. At this point, telomere shortening has been implicated in almost all aspects

The FDA Throws Up a Potential Roadblock

In his April 2010 column in *Forbes* magazine, Peter Huber pointed out the insanity of the Food and Drug Administration (FDA) regulations that currently block consideration of potential drugs to treat (that is, prevent or reverse) aging:

> For the most part, the FDA still operates under the medical mind-set that prevailed when the federal drug law was amended in 1962. The go/no-go regulatory calls are decided by clinical trials. The key metrics are clinical, like the survival time for a cancer patient. A clear reduction in mortality from a serious disease gets the drug licensed on the double. So far, so good—this panel sounds diligently anti-death. But it's interested only in brinkmanship, at the back end.
>
> The "aging" drugs that the FDA deals with reasonably well are the ones that beat back a single specific disease long after the microscopic seeds of the problem have blossomed into big symptoms. Aging is an incremental, whole-body problem. All cells, tissues and organs age—and in different ways, at different rates, in different people. As defined by their late-stage clinical symptoms, the diseases of old age are legion. At the FDA they will have to be beaten one at a time or not at all. Which means that nobody is ever going to get "antiaging" drugs through the FDA as it currently operates.

of normal aging. High levels of stress hormones, inflammation, insulin, and blood sugar, as well as habits and conditions such as smoking, fatty diets, obesity, and sedentary living, are all linked to shorter telomeres and lower telomerase levels. The conditions and diseases in which short telomeres are found include cancer, atherosclerosis, Alzheimer's disease, osteoarthritis, osteoporosis, macular degeneration, cirrhosis of the liver, AIDS, and even skin aging.

During the continuum of human life, the trillions of cells that make up a person continue to divide, grow, and replicate. With each cell division, a few base pairs at the tips of the chromosomes (telomeres) are lost, until the critical limit is reached. Then one of two things happens: the cell either enters senescence or commits suicide (apoptosis) and dies. In some people this process happens quickly; in others it can take much longer.

Cells die when telomeres become too short. Leonard Hayflick must have been correct after all—well, actually, no. While scientists were figuring out how telomeres function, they observed two interesting phenomena:

1. Telomere shortening proceeds at an uneven pace—the telomeres of some cells in the same group of cells become much shorter than others.
2. A few telomeres become longer. This was very surprising, because logically, telomere shortening should proceed at a steady pace, and telomeres should never get longer.

Something else was going on here. That something else was the biochemical catalyst, or enzyme, called *telomerase*. The discovery of telomerase was one of those wonderful moments in science history that belies the tediousness of most scientific research. Determined to prove their theory that indeed an enzyme did exist that caused telomere growth, Elizabeth Blackburn, then an ambitious molecular biologist at the University of California–Berkeley, and her second-year graduate student Carol Greider spent most of an entire year conducting failed experiments in which they tried to extract this particular enzyme from innumerable other enzymes in a crude cell extract. They were convinced that the enzyme they pursued was not ephemeral, but their first attempts required a complex process of purification and a long wait before results could be obtained. These efforts proved to be totally impractical.

Recalling these frustrating months, Greider says, "In the nine months I was doing this, I kept getting negative results. How much longer would I have gone on getting negative results before I would have decided, 'Well, it probably doesn't exist'?"

The breakthrough came after Blackburn decided to abandon the laboriously purified plasmid DNA fragments they were using for their experiments and instead try a synthetic and much more concentrated form of DNA called *oligonucleotides*. Within weeks, they obtained the results they had been looking for. On Christmas Day 1984, Greider developed an audioradiogram of their latest batch of DNA. Holding the X-ray image up to the light, she could see a clear pattern of recurring bands that extended like a ladder all the way up the gel. When Blackburn took a look, she noticed right away that the evenly spaced bands were too far apart to represent a random mix of DNA molecules. It was the proof they had been looking for: an enzyme had added telomeric DNA to the ends of the chromosomes.

Blackburn says about this moment, "Thoughts rushed through my mind that this discovery of a new enzymatic activity was as important as the discovery of DNA polymerase. DNA polymerase had garnered a Nobel Prize for its discoverer. I said nothing about this [to Greider], not wanting to raise unrealistic hopes. But we both knew this was it."

Blackburn and Greider had discovered the little enzyme that could. Many months later, they finally came up with a name for their discovery. They called the enzyme *telomerase*.

Although it would be years before the full significance of telomerase was truly appreciated, we now know that it is present and active in both germ cells and cancer cells, which is one of several reasons these cells never reach senescence. The telomerase gene also exists in all our other cells, because the DNA in every one of our cells is identical—a stem cell, a muscle cell, and

The Cancer Question

In addition to telomerase providing a way to counter the aging of cells, extensive research into the enzyme has given us many new insights into cancer and its prevention. It is possible to cause cancer cells to die by turning off or inhibiting telomerase, which is giving rise to a whole new class of drugs called *telomerase inhibitors*. Overactivation of telomerase is one of the few constants between almost all types of cancers; it is present in 85% of all cancer cells, whether breast cancer, lung cancer, prostate cancer, or any other cancer. Instead of trying to create dozens of therapies for dozens of different cancers, we could very well be looking at one type of therapy for all types of cancers.

Lest anyone be confused, however, it is important to point out that stimulating the growth of telomeres on normal chromosomes does not cause them to become cancerous. A cancer begins when something else goes wrong in a cell, causing it to lose control over its growth. However, the telomeres continue to shorten in these cells, and very soon these fast-dividing cancer cells will die.

Very occasionally, however, they will find ways to turn on the telomerase gene and relengthen their telomeres. When this happens, a cancer begins to divide not only uncontrollably but also indefinitely. The cancer becomes truly dangerous.

So, turning on the telomerase of normal cells must be highly dangerous, right?

The answer to this question is a resounding *no*. Although telomerase is necessary for cancers to extend their life span, it does not cause cancer. This fact has been repeatedly demonstrated by performing many different types of genetic tests for cancer on telomerase-positive human cells. Scientists have turned on the telomerase of normal cells in attempts to turn these cells into cancer cells, and it just hasn't happened.

Generally speaking, bad things happen when telomeres become short. As cells approach senescence, the short telomeres stimulate chromosome instability, which can cause the mutations that cause cancer. Tumor-suppressor genes can be shut off and cancer-causing genes turned on. The result becomes very dangerous if another mutation causes telomerase to be turned on.

Paradoxically, even though cells require telomerase to become dangerous cancers, turning on telomerase may actually prevent cancer. This is not just because the risk of chromosome rearrangements is reduced, but also because telomerase can extend the life span of our immune cells, improving their ability to seek and destroy cancer cells.

If long telomeres in human beings were correlated with cancer, young people would get cancer more often than the elderly do. However, we usually see cancers occurring in people at the same time they begin to show signs of cellular senescence—that is, at the same time the immune system begins to age and lose its ability to respond to threats. According to the American Cancer Society, 78 percent of all cancers are diagnosed in people fifty-eight years old and older. Extending the life span of our immune cells could help our bodies fight cancer for much longer than they presently do.

a liver cell contain exactly the same genetic information. The crucial difference is that normal cells don't express telomerase, because that gene is repressed in them. The key to immortality is turning the telomerase gene from off to on.

In 1997, scientists inserted active telomerase genes into human skin cells grown in a petri dish. When they observed that the telomerase enzyme was being produced in the cells, as they had hoped it would be, they also observed that the skin cells became immortal. There was no limit to the number of times these cells could divide. Better yet, when the lengths of these telomerized cells were examined, the scientists were surprised to see that the telomeres didn't just stop shortening, they actually grew longer. The critical question, at the time unanswered, was whether the cells were becoming younger.

A few years later, scientists inserted the telomerase gene into human skin cells that already had very short telomeres. These cells were then grown into skin on the back of mice. As you might expect, the skin from cells that hadn't received the telomerase gene looked like old skin. It was wrinkled, it blistered easily, and it had gene expression patterns indicative of old skin.

The skin grown from cells that had received the telomerase gene, in contrast, looked young. It acted like young skin, and its gene expression patterns were almost identical to the gene expression patterns of young skin. For the first time, scientists had demonstrably reversed aging in human cells.

A Parts Supply Store for the Human Body

On March 16, 2010, the stock of BioTime, a small biotechnology company in Alameda, California, soared upon the news that the company had induced normal adult human cells not only to reverse their age but also to reverse what is called their *clock of differentiation*. That is, the age of these cells was reversed to the extent that they went all the way back in time to their original state as stem cells. Because stem cells are capable of being regenerated into any type of human cells, this suggests therapies for regrowing heart cells, skin cells, muscle cells, and so on, without having to resort to the highly controversial practice of using embryonic stem cells.

"We are just at the beginning of some really fascinating new possibilities for intervening in age-related disease," said BioTime's CEO, Michael West. "What's exciting about these cells is we now have a way to simply have a master cell bank of the stem cells and

Why Are We Not Born Old?

Reproductive cells are considered immortal by scientists. This means that they do not age in the normal way that other cells do. Sperm cells divide millions of times, and their telomeres never get short. In sperm cells, the enzyme telomerase adds telomere DNA back to the cells' telomeres and keeps those telomeres as long as they have always been. That's why an eighty-year-old man can still father children. Egg cells, on the other hand, do not divide, and therefore their telomeres do not shorten.

In addition to providing the germ cell with an unending ability to reproduce itself, telomerase also generally keeps the DNA tightly wound (not unraveled), so the cell is not subject to the normal wear and tear that other cells in the body are subjected to.

Thus, reproductive cells do not lose telomere length as we age, and accordingly, babies are born with telomeres the length of babies' and not the length of their parents'. Ultimately, if it were not for telomerase keeping germ cells young, a species would become extinct.

scalably make everything of the human body—like a human parts supply store."

Just imagine: if your knees wear out, it will someday, in the not-too-distant future, be possible to replace them with real knees rather than artificial ones, and they will be genetically identical to your original knees because they will be able to be grown from your own stem cells!

Biomedical scientist Robert Schwartz from the University of Houston has already demonstrated how to grow human heart cells from adult stem cells that have been harvested from a patient's own skin. These new cells can be implanted and grown into fully developed beating heart cells, and they will reverse the damage caused by previous heart attacks by replacing the damaged cardiac tissue. So far this work has been done in vitro, but clinical trials using these programmed cells on actual heart patients will begin within a year or two.

Schwartz's vision is similar to Michael West's, only he expresses it differently: "The idea of having your own bag of stem cells that you can carry through life and use for tissue regeneration is at the very cutting edge of science."

New brain cells will someday be used to treat Alzheimer's patients and people with severe brain trauma, or a diabetic could get new insulin-producing cells in the pancreas. Generating a new kidney, lung, or liver will also be possible—even an entire new heart! But we have an even loftier goal in creating the Immortality Edge program. We want to give you the possibility of being forever young so that your body doesn't wear out or become disease-ridden. If you can keep your telomeres long enough, and even grow them to be longer, you will never have to face the deterioration of getting old. You'll instead remain forever young.

How Will the Earth Hold Us All?

One of the first questions that invariably comes up during discussions of life extension or anti-aging strategies is "What will we do with all the people?"

It stands to reason that life extension and immortality would increase the world population; after all, we've seen it happen before. In just over a century, the average life expectancy of a person living in the United States has increased from 47.3 years in 1900 to 78 years in 2008. Technologies—including vaccines, antibiotics, chemotherapy, and antioxidants—as well as social advances such as sanitation, environmentalism, and an antismoking crusade have all contributed to this. Most recently, we've made attempts to push our life expectancy even further with technologies such as hormone replacement, caloric restriction.

These technologies have indeed increased the size of our population. But something interesting also happened: the population growth rate began to slow down. Birthrates fell rapidly, and in less than four decades, the average number of children in a family in the United States was more than cut in half, from 6 to 2.9. Today, most leading population researchers think that the world is headed quickly toward a stable population. Evidence is mounting that humans will simply not reach populations larger than our ability to sustain them; economics precludes us from doing that. As resources become scarce, prices rise, and as prices rise, family sizes shrink.

Is it a bad thing that our medical advances have nearly doubled our life expectancy? Most would say it's a decidedly good thing. So it's probably a safe bet that if we can drastically increase that figure again, future generations will also look back on it as beneficial.

Let's be realistic, too, about how many people will take the time to understand the telomere biology in this book and adopt the strategies we recommend for slowing down or even reversing telomere shortening. Unless *The Immortality Edge* outsells the Bible, we don't have much to worry about.

If tomorrow morning the scientists at Sierra Sciences, a company based in Reno, Nevada, that searches for telomerase inducers, announce that they have found the perfect compound for switching on telomerase, how long will it take to get this compound developed into a drug, tested, approved by the FDA, and put into the marketplace in large enough quantities to make much of a statistical difference in world population?

How many people even want to live an indefinite life span? We think it is sad that most people accept death as inevitable, and it will be a very long time before the majority realizes that this is no longer the only option.

Death Is Not Inevitable

Each of us carries within the self a unique and complex universe of knowledge, skills, wisdom, life experiences, and human relationships. Almost all of this rich treasury of information is forever lost when someone dies. As famed neuroscientist Anders Sandberg likes to point out, "Every time a human being dies, a library burns. It is a horrible tragedy that all our life experiences get lost, both the good and the bad." It is worth stating again and again: death is not inevitable.

"In the same way we have one-hundred-year-old cars that are working just as well as they did when they rolled off the production line," says Aubrey de Grey, the Oxford biogerontologist who is often considered the leader of the entire anti-aging movement, "once we are able to implement comprehensive repair [and] maintenance technologies, we'll be able to do the same for the human body. The first human being to live to one thousand is already among us."

If you believe that you have no purpose in life and nothing much to contribute to other people, then this book is not for you. However, if you love living and still have many things you would like to accomplish, then living as long as possible will let you achieve more and become a more valuable person. You'll have time, metaphorically speaking, to build the city of Rome all by yourself!

What could be better than this? What do you have to do to live as long as you want? As you'll soon discover by reading *The Immortality Edge*, there are many ways to keep your telomeres long and healthy. You can start today by eating telomere-friendly foods, exercising the right way, meditating, taking supplements that have been linked to longer telomeres, and making some other lifestyle changes we recommend. There is even a pill you can take that has been proven to lengthen telomeres. It's all right here.

If you let us help you stay healthy, vital, and young for only an extra ten to twenty years, we have no doubt whatsoever that new medical therapies (for example, regenerative medicine) and new supplements will be available that will not just slow telomere shortening but will reverse it. It will actually be possible for you to become biologically younger and to live indefinitely.

For the winter holiday season of 2084, we plan to organize a celebration on the Island of Fiji to celebrate the one-hundredth anniversary of Elizabeth Blackburn and Carol Greider's discovery of telomerase; incidentally, this will also be the seventy-fourth anniversary of the publication of this book. By reading *The Immortality Edge*, you're automatically invited to join us and be part of the first significant group of human beings to blast through the Hayflick limit.

We hope to see you there.

The Quick Telomere Age Test

This test will give you a rough idea of what your telomere age is. For a more accurate result, take the complete test in chapter 5.

Start with your chronological age and add or subtract from it based on the answers to the following questions:

1. Do you exercise for at least forty-five minutes three or more times a week? If yes, subtract five years.
2. Do you smoke cigarettes? Add ten years.
3. Do you currently drink three or more drinks of alcohol on a daily basis? Add seven years.
4. Do you sleep between seven and nine hours most nights? Subtract five years.

5. If you are male and your waist is less than thirty-six inches, subtract five years. If you are female and your waist is less than thirty-two inches, likewise, subtract five years.
6. Do you take fish oil? If you take 3,000 milligrams a day or more, subtract five years.
7. Generally speaking, are you happy? Subtract seven years.
8. Do you eat fried foods more than twice a week? Add three years.

PART ONE

The Immortality Promise

1

The Aging Cure

Is aging a disease or a natural process that has existed forever? You may be surprised to learn that aging has not existed forever. Approximately four and a half billion years ago, a single cell came into existence that was the progenitor of every living organism that has existed on our planet ever since. This single cell did not age; it had the capacity to divide indefinitely. It could produce an infinite number of copies of itself, and it would not die until some outside environmental event, such as an erupting volcano, killed it.

The ancestry of every living cell in your body can be traced back to this very first cell. This lineage is called the cell's *germ line*.

Three billion years after the first cell appeared, some of the cells from this germ line began to form multicellular organisms, such as worms, insects, fish, and finally humans. The germ line was passed from one generation to the next, and it remained immortal. Even with the inclusion of multicellular organisms, the germ line itself showed no signs of aging.

However, the cells that form the body of an organism, called *somatic cells*, began to age. Their ability to reproduce themselves indefinitely came to an end. Until recently, scientists were only able to speculate why somatic cells die.

We now know why. Unlike germ cells, somatic cells contain a gene that controls the production of telomerase, and this gene is turned off. Without the ability to produce telomerase (except in trace amounts), the telomeres of somatic cells become shorter and shorter with each replication, until the cell finally goes into senescence and dies.

The speed at which our telomeres shorten is determined by the outcome of the endless war our organism wages on the damaging forces that actively attempt to destroy our molecules, our cells, and our entire bodies. At every moment we are engaged in an internal struggle against negative forces, including oxidation, glycation (described later), inflammation, DNA gene mutation, and abnormal methylation (described later). Simultaneously, we are also dealing with external threats: environmental toxins, natural catastrophes, war, and other forms of violence. When we lose any of these battles at any level—biochemical, cellular, systemic, or in the whole organism—death can and does occur.

At every level, life is a balance between entropy and defense, degradation and restoration. Our bodies are miraculously designed to defend us from any attack. At every level, we have specific ways of minimizing, avoiding, replacing, and repairing damage.

As you mature into an adult human being, at some point, usually around age forty, your body is no longer able to build new proteins as quickly as it loses them. You can synthesize them as accurately as before, but there are also more damaged proteins, because they don't recycle as fast as they did when you were younger. As a result, the damaged proteins linger. It's not that there are fewer proteins to go around; it's just that the turnover slows down. Protein synthesis declines by more than half, and so does protein breakdown. Our cells don't recycle as well as they once did, and as a result, the number of damaged proteins in our bodies at any given time increases. As the balance shifts toward the forces of decay, we age faster. Age-related defects in metabolism add to pathology. The pace of telomere shortening picks up.

The aging process we are describing here is strikingly similar to what happens when our bodies develop specific diseases, including Alzheimer's disease, diabetes, cardiovascular disease, and even cancer. The core cause of type 2 diabetes, for example, is a gradual decline in the number of beta cells in the pancreas. These beta cells make and release insulin. Alzheimer's disease is

---

How We've Extended Life Expectancy

Since 1900, the average life expectancy in the United States has risen nearly 60 percent, from 47.3 years to 78 years. The following is a list of factors that account for much, if not most, of this improvement:

Antibiotics
Antioxidants
Better diets
Better teeth and gum hygiene
Blood pressure medicine
Cleaner water
Coronary artery bypass surgery
Hormone replacement
Improved management of hazardous chemicals
Improved public awareness of nutrition
Improved sewage systems
Medications that improve vascular health
More effective cancer treatments
More exercise
Reduced smoking
Refrigeration
Some vaccines

associated with an accumulation of amyloid plaques (an abnormal protein breakdown product that interferes with normal cell function, among other processes) and tangles in the brain. Heart disease is associated with the buildup of fatty plaques and the gradual hardening of the arteries. And cancer, of course, is associated with the growth of malignant cells.

Old age underlies most diseases. We believe that old age actually *is* a disease and it simply has many faces. Each disease is individual and separate from all others, yet the erosion of the telomere plays a role in all diseases of aging. One disease can hasten another. If the telomere did not shorten, most diseases would have a different appearance, and a few might not appear at all. In recent years, overwhelming evidence has emerged that genetic and lifestyle interventions, in parallel, can retard nearly all late-life disease. And guess what: these lifestyle interventions also slow down aging.

The belief that aging is an immutable process, programmed by evolution, is simply wrong. Aging is a disease, and just as we do with other diseases, we should create drugs and other technologies to cure it. The mere fact that aging has existed in the genetic code for roughly one billion years doesn't change this. Thousands of other diseases, from hemophilia to cystic fibrosis, have lurked in our genes for far longer than recorded history.

Immortality Is Just around the Corner

Do we currently have the knowledge and the technologies to live forever? At this precise moment in time, the answer would have to be no. We can dramatically slow down diseases and the aging process far more than most people realize, but we do not yet have the "magic bullet" to indefinitely extend human life.

We now know, however, what the solution most likely will be, and there is every reason to believe that it will be available sometime in the next twenty years. It will be a drug therapy that turns on the telomerase gene in healthy somatic cells.

At least one biotechnology company we are familiar with, Sierra Sciences in Reno, Nevada, is completely devoted to discovering chemical compounds that, as the company describes it, induce telomerase gene activity in normal human cells without killing them. Sierra Sciences found its first telomerase inducer on November 6, 2007, and as of this writing, the company has screened more than 250,000 compounds and found 38 different chemicals that induce telomerase expression. The most potent of these, however, is only 12 percent of what they believe they need to make a human cell immortal. Sierra Sciences is currently screening 4,000 compounds a week.

Another company, T. A. Sciences, Inc., in New York City, has a supplement in pill form that it claims has been lab tested and shown to turn on telomerase and lengthen the shortest telomeres. This is critically important because it only takes one short telomere to send a cell into crisis. This product, TA-65, contains a single molecule of the astragalus plant, which has been used in Chinese medicine for thousands of years, often in combination with other herbs, to strengthen the body's immune system. The company purifies the rare (expensive!) substance through an extensive process, which also factors into its high price, from $2,400 to $8,000 per year.

The efficacy of TA-65 is incremental. It does seem to stop telomere shortening and minutely lengthen telomeres, but not in the profound way that future drugs will. One natural compound that may prove more powerful and more affordable may be available by the time this book is published. You can find updates on it at www.maxlife.org/telomeres. Still, TA-65 is currently being used by the authors of this book, and Dr. Woynarowski is one of the physicians who is licensed to distribute it.

Living Long Enough to Live Forever

The telomere theory of aging, though it is gaining traction, is not the only theory of what causes aging. Because aging is not a simple process and may indeed have multiple causes, there are quite a few feasible ideas floating about. Here's a short list.

Other Theories on the Cause of Aging

* *Disposable soma.* We are just a temporary house for our genes. At some point, our genes get tired of us and move out.
* *Free radicals.* Free radicals cause mutations in our proteins and our DNA. When enough free-radical damage accumulates, we die.
* *Vital substance.* We have a limited amount of some undiscovered vital substance.
* *Gene mutation.* The accumulation of mutations causes aging. This ties into the free-radical theory above.
* *Reproductive exhaustion.* After a burst of reproductive activity, a switch is flipped. We die rapidly.
* *Aging by design.* We are simply programmed to die.
* *Wear and tear.* Aubrey de Grey, an Oxford biogerontologist, likens the aging process to an old car, where our body parts simply wear out over time.
* *Waste-product accumulation.* Like a clogged water filter with too much debris, our cells and bodies no longer function as they should.
* *Cross-linkage.* A process called *glycation* causes sugar molecules to bind with protein molecules, creating globs of gunk called *advanced glycation end products* (AGEs). These build up, causing diseases that age us and eventually kill us.
* *Immune system.* The decreased efficiency of the immune system causes aging.
* *Errors of repairs.* The inaccurate repair of cellular damage causes aging.
* *Order to disorder.* A decrease occurs in the efficiency of the systems *that maintain order. Things* get messed up, we age, they get more messed up, and we die.

One thing all of these theories have in common is that they are all related to accelerated telomere loss and damage.

But just as the telomere theory of aging isn't the only theory, telomerase activation isn't the only proposed method for obtaining an infinite life span. One intriguing idea comes from nanomedicine, a branch of nanotechnology. The idea is to create microscopic machines to be sent on missions inside our bodies to inspect, repair, and reconstruct cells.

Nanomedicine theorist Robert Freitas, who is the senior research fellow at the Institute of Molecular Manufacturing in Palo Alto, California, points out that if "the idea of placing millions of autonomous nanobots inside one's body might seem odd, even alarming, the fact is that the body already teems with a vast number of mobile nanodevices." In other words, biology itself provides the proof that nanomedicine is feasible.

We are quite positive that the cause of and the solution to aging lies in telomere biology. If we are wrong, and it lies elsewhere, what difference will it make, as long as you are still around to benefit from another solution? The more important question is "What will it take to keep you alive long enough?"

Aubrey de Grey, the Oxford biogerontologist we quoted earlier about hundred-year-old cars, says, "The people who are working on [these cars] aren't doing any more sophisticated work on them now than they were doing fifty years ago, when the cars were only three or four times as old as they were designed to be. When you decide to do sufficiently comprehensive maintenance, that's it. You can keep the machine at a manageable level of damage, a level that is not prejudicial to the functioning of the machine."

De Grey has a point. Mechanical maintenance of your body will help to keep it running. There is an important difference, however, between cars and humans. Unlike cars, our bodies contain hidden destructive forces. If these forces are not counteracted, they can cause you to age even faster than normal. Identifying and controlling them is central to your battle to keep your telomeres as long as possible for as long as possible.

If we could remove the genetic factor from aging and disease, we would still be left with about 70 percent of the real causes. According to the Human Genome Project, 30 percent of what happens to us is determined by our genes and inheritance; the other 70 percent is determined by our environment and how well we maintain ourselves (like the vintage automobiles). That's good news; it means that maintenance gives us two-to-one odds that we can influence our future health in a very positive way.

To understand aging and illness as well as more subtle problems like sexual dysfunction, brain fog, fatigue, and weakness, you need to penetrate to the level of the individual cell. You also have to keep a kind of biological flowchart in mind: cells form tissues, tissues form organs, organs form organ systems, and organ systems form organisms (you and us!) when they operate in synchronized fashion. You are only as good as your weakest link (which might just be your shortest telomeres!), so even a small population of dysfunctional cells can put a big load on the rest of your body, ultimately leading to sickness and death.

The Major Aging Factors

At the cellular level as well as at higher levels, three major aging factors—oxidation, inflammation, and glycation—can wreak havoc in our bodies. They work in concert, feed upon one another, and make one another stronger and far more deadly. Abnormal methylation is also a factor in aging.

Showing you how to minimize the impact of these aging factors is a major purpose of this book. We want you to defeat oxidation, inflammation, glycation, and abnormal methylation so that you can extend both your health span and your life span. We want you to be available for the even more potent anti-aging telomere therapy that is bound to come along in the near future.

Oxidation

The first aging factor, oxidation, is represented by free radicals, high-energy molecules that are unstable because each has a single, unpaired electron in its outermost shell. This electron is essentially homeless; it keeps trying to find a partner, even when that means stealing an electron from, and damaging, other molecules. Free radicals roam about our bodies with haphazard abandon, interfering with normal cell function. Like molecular sharks, they are constantly hungry, latching on to almost any nearby molecule, damaging it by changing its shape and making it useless or even dangerous. The damaged molecule becomes a misshapen, crippled player on the molecular team. Not only does it no longer function by itself, it interferes with the functioning of its surrounding teammates.

In this way, free radicals are infectious, passing on their unpaired electrons to other victims, which then pass on electrons that become the source of further damage. The chain of damage extends indefinitely and terminates only when the single electron finds a suitable mate and at last settles down and is once again at peace.

Ironically, the most common free radical in your body is oxygen, an element you cannot live without. Although molecular oxygen is relatively stable, it takes only a very small energy fluctuation to form single oxygen atoms, which are remarkably reactive with other molecules. The damage that single oxygen atoms do is specific, depending on exactly which free radical gets loose—the solubility, acidity, and proximity to specific sites all determine what is damaged.

As you age, free-radical damage to your DNA increases. Certain areas of your DNA are especially vulnerable to free-radical damage. This is important because there are only limited amounts of DNA available, the repair mechanisms are not perfect, and DNA is the blueprint for all other molecules in your body.

Countering the effects of these free radicals are "reduction molecules" that function like free radical "sponges" soaking up excess energy without being damaged themselves or causing damage to other cells. This balance is a critical part of cellular biochemistry. Only when the situation becomes unbalanced do problems occur and you have what is called *oxidative stress*. This happens when there are too many free radicals or relatively not enough reduction molecules, or when the regenerative and repair machinery of the cell is too sick or old to keep up with free-radical generation and is unable to neutralize it.

As you'll see in the chapters on supplements and nutrition (chapters 2 and 6, respectively) there are many ways to decrease the production of free radicals and thereby minimize the damage to your telomere segments as well as the rest of the cell. In general, these supplement and food choices will also benefit the health of your mitochondria, the engine inside cells where energy is burned and where free radicals originate. In chapter 2 you will learn a great deal about mitochondria.

Inflammation

The second aging factor is inflammation. Only a decade ago, inflammatory diseases were believed to be confined to conditions with obvious, or acute, inflammation, such as the inflamed joints of arthritis, the inflamed airways of asthma, or even the inflamed skin of acne. Since then, however, a chronic, or silent, inflammation has been discovered to play a main role in diseases that had not been considered inflammatory at all, including heart disease and other vascular diseases, Alzheimer's disease, diabetes, and certain types of cancer. The symptoms of chronic inflammation are altogether different from the symptoms of acute inflammation. Chronic inflammation is hardly noticeable until catastrophe strikes.

Chronic low-grade inflammation can smolder silently within your body for twenty or thirty years and even longer without causing any obvious or outward problems. But all that time it is eroding your health and taking years from your life.

Cardiologists once thought that heart disease was caused simply by the buildup of cholesterol deposits inside the walls of the coronary arteries. Now we know that chronic inflammation is a fundamental reason for cholesterol being deposited in the arteries in the first place.

We know that chronic inflammation is also at the root of Alzheimer's disease. In the brain, it increases the production of soluble amyloid protein and increases its conversion into insoluble amyloid fibrils, which are toxic waste products that interfere with normal brain functioning and kill brain cells.

In type 2 diabetes, chronic inflammation is behind the formation of a different type of amyloid that forms in the pancreas. The chronic elevation of blood sugar and insulin levels increases inflammation in the bloodstream, triggering a cascade of events in the pancreas of type 2 diabetes patients similar to what is seen in the brain of an Alzheimer's patient.

Although it is premature to come out and flatly say that inflammation is the primary cause of all nongenetic diseases and of aging, it certainly plays a major role.

Chronic inflammation affects the telomeres as well, causing them to shorten at a faster than normal rate. Recent research seems to indicate that there may be tissue-specific telomere shortening in many diseases. People with heart disease, for instance, may have shorter telomeres in their heart tissues than in other places. People with Alzheimer's disease appear to have a disproportionate shortening of their brain telomeres.

Like many things, the amount of inflammation in your body is largely under your own control. You can reduce inflammation by eating more vegetables and, in particular, medium- and low-glycemic fruits for their antioxidant value, increasing your fish or fish oil consumption, getting a decent amount of the right kind of exercise, improving your stress response, and sleeping better. Importantly, as you will learn in our chapter on nutrition, there is an eating plan based on the age-old trends of hunter-gatherers that we, along with some top evolutionary scientists and researchers, believe can naturally reduce inflammation by matching your nutritional genetics with what you eat. This plan is called the Paleolithic Diet.

The nutrition, exercise, and stress reduction sections of this book are all keyed toward helping you to lower your inflammation levels.

Glycation

Glycation is the third aging factor. You may not realize it, but there's a double-edged sword hiding in seemingly harmless foods such as bread, salad dressing, fruit juice, ketchup, mustard, and some brands of tomato sauce, to name a few. All of these everyday consumables could be contributing to the slow and steady destruction of your cellular health, thanks to one dangerous ingredient: sugar. The odds are that sugar is sabotaging your health and making you age faster right now, at this very moment.

When your body is exposed to too much sugar, including too many carbohydrates that convert to sugar when you eat them, the process of glycation is triggered: the sugar molecules attach themselves to the molecules of proteins and fats (lipids). The result is

---

Basic Sugars and Sweeteners

Are you confused by all of the different sugars and sweeteners? It's no wonder, because there are so many of them. This list should help you to sort it out:

- *Dextrose, fructose, and glucose.* All are monosaccharides, or simple sugars; the difference lies in how your body metabolizes them. Dextrose and glucose are essentially the same; however, food manufacturers usually use *dextrose* on their nutrition labels.
- *Table sugar.* Half glucose and half fructose, disaccharide, or table sugar, is a complex sugar formed from two simple sugars.

- *High fructose corn syrup (HFCS)*. HFCS, which is 55 percent fructose and 45 percent glucose, may well be the most damaging of all sugars. You can trace the rise of diabetes in the United States with the increased use of this corn-based product. It is everywhere, including in most sodas and even in some breads.
- *Ethanol*. The form of alcohol that is in alcoholic drinks, ethanol is not a sugar, although beer and wine contain residual sugars and starches.
- *Sugar alcohols*. Examples are xylitol, glycerol, sorbitol, maltitol, mannitol, and erythritol. These are neither sugars nor alcohols but are becoming increasingly popular as sweeteners. They are incompletely absorbed in your small intestine, so they provide fewer calories than sugar but often cause bloating, diarrhea, and flatulence.
- *Sucralose (Splenda)*. This is not a sugar, despite its sugar-like name and the deceptive marketing slogan "made from sugar." Splenda is a chlorinated artificial sweetener in line with aspartame and saccharin, with detrimental health effects to match.
- *Agave syrup*. Falsely advertised as "natural," agave syrup is highly processed and is usually 80 percent fructose. It does not even remotely resemble the original agave plant.
- *Honey*. Honey is about 53 percent fructose, but in its raw form it is completely natural and has health benefits, including antioxidants, when used in moderation.
- *Stevia*. This is a very sweet herb derived from the leaf of the South American stevia plant, which is completely safe. This does not raise your blood sugar, and many people like its taste.

called *cross linkages*. The molecules involved become damaged, the cell membranes become less elastic, and some cells die.

The result of glycation, as noted earlier, is the formation of clumps called AGEs. Over time, AGEs accumulate throughout your body, triggering chronic inflammation and damaging just about every tissue. Think of it this way: if you took a sugared soda, poured it on the floor, and let it dry without wiping it up, you'd have a sticky mess. The same thing happens inside your cells when AGEs are formed.

AGEs trigger the abnormal clumping of blood platelets, which causes the blood vessels to narrow and thereby contributes to high blood pressure, vascular disease, and heart attacks. AGEs are also linked to insulin resistance, poor blood sugar control, and the accumulation of damaging amyloid substances in the brain. The more we learn about AGEs, the more we realize that they are implicated in a whole range of diseases, including rheumatoid arthritis, kidney disease, inflammatory bowel disorders such as colitis, and inflammatory skin conditions such as eczema. They can even damage your eyes.

You can reduce the number of AGEs in your system by cutting back on sugars, avoiding simple (as opposed to complex) carbohydrates, learning how to detect hidden sugars in processed foods, and avoiding food that has been browned by high-temperature overcooking. Most of our food has some sugar in it, and overcooking (including microwaving) a food causes the sugar to caramelize, which results when foods form AGEs.

In a study published by the *Journal of Clinical Endocrinology and Metabolism* while we were writing this book, researchers from the National Institute on Aging and the Mount Sinai School of Medicine divided forty healthy participants and nine participants with kidney disease into two groups. One group ate a normal, high-AGE diet, and the other group reduced AGE intake by half by avoiding high-temperature cooking. The groups' caloric and nutrient intake were identical. After four months, the low-AGE group—including those with kidney disease—showed dramatic improvements in markers of inflammation and in blood-vessel health. To cut down on AGEs, the researchers advised "keeping the heat down and the water content up in food and avoiding pre-packaged and fast foods." Meat eaters may wish to avoid well-done meat.

We agree! Since AGEs have such devastating consequences, anyone would be wise to limit their intake as much as possible.

Abnormal Methylation

Abnormal methylation is another aging factor. Methylation is a simple chemical process in which a methyl group (one carbon atom and three hydrogen atoms) becomes attached to other molecules. It is generally a good thing. Your body uses methylation to help rid itself of a number of dangerous heavy metal toxins. The liver uses methylation to assist in the excretion of external toxins such as pesticides as well as some of its own chemical wastes, such as hormone by-products. Methylation reactions are also critical to normal brain function.

Methylation controls the expression of genes in the body, silencing the bad ones and letting the good ones be "read." It also stabilizes the telomere segments, protecting them from loss due to oxidation, and it may be the reaction that turns on telomerase, the only currently known safe and natural way to lengthen your telomeres.

Unfortunately, depending on age and ethnicity, 10 to 44 percent of people in the United States have abnormal methylation, which can lead to cervical cancer, colon cancer, heart disease, stroke, Alzheimer's disease, and other bad conditions.

No one is sure what causes this, but the good news is that at least one form of abnormal methylation is easy to detect with a simple blood test that measures a chemical in your body called homocysteine. Homocysteine is an inflammatory compound formed by abnormal protein metabolism. Your body can use the methylation process to reduce toxic levels of homocysteine.

In a healthy person, this happens quite easily, but if your methylation is abnormal, homocysteine accumulates to toxic levels. High levels of homocysteine are linked to heart attack, stroke, and atherosclerosis.

If a blood test finds that your homocysteine levels are high, you can reduce them by taking vitamin B supplements, including a larger than normal dose of folic acid, up to 10,000 micrograms per day.

You can help your body to effectively methylate by some of the means we have already discussed and by others we will discuss in subsequent chapters. The choice of foods—mainly vegetables and fruits of a low to moderate glycemic index—gives you a potent dose of antioxidants that aids the methylation process. The proper choice of foods (see chapter 6) also decreases the acid load your body has to deal with and leads to a more favorable methylation environment.

The Lucrative Side of Longevity

If aging is a disease, it must be the mother of all diseases. If we can find a way to intervene against the entropic forces, to slow down or even reverse the accumulation of damaged proteins, we will be on the path to curing not only aging but also all of the diseases associated with aging. We will also realize what enlightened biogerontologists and other scientists who study aging call the *longevity dividend*.

The longevity dividend, first proposed in an article published in the *Scientist* in March 2006, means that in addition to the obvious health benefits, enormous economic good will accrue from the extension of healthy life. Billions will be saved in future health-care expenses, because people who are sick less often and for shorter periods of time will cost the economy much less. Also, by extending the amount of time in the average life span in which higher levels of physical and mental capacity are expressed, many people will remain in the workforce longer, personal income and savings will increase, and age-entitlement programs will face less pressure from shifting demographics.

Instead of longevity causing us to succumb to bankruptcy, as conventional wisdom would have us believe, national economies will flourish.

The article in the *Scientist* explains, "If we succeed in slowing aging by seven years, the age-specific risk of death, frailty, and disability will be reduced by approximately half at every age. People who reach the age of 50 in the future would have the health profile and disease risk of today's 43-year-old; those age 60 would resemble current 53-year-olds, and so on."

Slowing down aging enough to delay death by seven years, while laudable, is for us an extremely conservative goal. If you are willing to make the lifestyle changes, follow the fitness and nutritional guides, and take up the meditation that we recommend, you should be able to extend your life span and your health span much longer than this—long enough, in fact, to take advantage of therapies that will activate the telomere gene in your somatic cells. This will cause your telomeres to grow and biologically reverse your aging process. Even as you become chronologically older, you will, in fact, become biologically younger.

We suggest that, given the scientific nature of much of what you will be reading, you break this book into manageable sections and take a break as needed, but that you begin the nutritional, exercise, and stress-reduction sections as soon as possible. That way your body will be able to begin turning back the clock as your mind gets up to speed. Once you have fully digested the science behind our program, you will be even more motivated to continue and pleased that you have already begun to do the good work involved in getting more youthful, not older, as time goes on.

PART TWO

The Immortality Edge
Longevity Program

2

The Immortality Edge
Supplement Plan

In an ideal world, we would all eat well all the time. Our food would not be grown in nutrient-poor soil that contains pesticides and heavy metals from acid rain. Cattle, chickens, and other animals wouldn't be raised in unsanitary conditions, pumped full of hormones and antibiotics. Produce wouldn't be cleaned and packaged in huge factorylike warehouses where *E. coli* and other bacteria can quickly spread and become untraceable—an unfortunate by-product of mass production that is known to contaminate even organic food.

Even if the food we ate were as pure as the water in an ancient glacier, it still couldn't provide the optimal amount of specific nutrients, so to protect our telomeres we must push our first defense to high alert. For example, which would you rather do to get the optimal amount of phytonutrients to fortify your immune system: eat five pounds of broccoli followed by a quart of blueberries, or take a well-crafted supplement that delivers the equivalent power?

Even though our food is not as good as it was only a century ago, you should still make every effort to eat right. The wholesome foods we recommend provide fiber and the natural proportions of vitamins and minerals that your body can recognize and use effectively. Following our nutrition plan will reduce oxidative stress and the resulting inflammation that is known to speed up telomere shortening.

The unfortunate truth is that unless you are a saint, you are like everyone else, and everyone else slips up once in a while, eating some french fries or having a double-chocolate mocha with whipped cream, if not something far worse. And guess what: the effects of pollution, radiation, and toxins in the environment, combined with the stress of sleep deprivation or everyday irritations, do not stop just because you're on the latest macrobiotic diet.

The bottom line is that no matter what some nutritionists may say, depending solely on food for your nutritional needs is not enough. If you want to live as long as possible while maintaining your vitality—if you want to keep your telomeres from shrinking

A Guide to Buying Supplements

Not all supplements are the same. As we were writing this, a lawsuit was filed in California against nine companies that market fish oil for not revealing that their products contain toxic levels of PCBs above the allowable amounts. One of these companies is a large chain of pharmacies, so it's not just the "mom and pop" enterprises you need to look out for. Because we want you to use supplements, we urge you to follow these guidelines:

- Buy products with only the highest-quality ingredients. You may pay more for these, just as you would for a better car, computer, or meal, but like these things, supplements are worth it. Inferior ingredients in supplements can be contaminated, improperly formulated, and hard to digest, and in some cases they can do more harm than good.

- Look for brands that deliver third-party independent testing of their products, including purity, on a frequent basis.
- Buy from companies that have a long record of success in the supplement industry. Lousy supplements do not survive in the highly competitive and crowded supplement industry. For every vitamin or mineral you see in a pharmacy or a vitamin store, there are ten other brands that never made it or that failed.
- Be leery of buzzwords and marketing labels. Educate yourself to know some of the research behind specific nutraceuticals so you won't fall victim to false and exaggerated claims. When using the Internet to validate scientific claims, be very aware of the source. Did the "facts" in the article you're reading come from a prestigious university like Harvard or Stanford, or did they come from a "study" funded by the company that makes the supplement? Look for product descriptions and related online information that you can understand.
- Beware of private-label supplements. The vast majority of supplements are made by the consumer divisions of big pharmaceutical companies, then relabeled into many different brands by the distributors. For example, Dr. Schmoker's One-a-Day may just be a repackaged version of a cheaply mass-manufactured standard multivitamin with the good doctor's mug plastered on the bottle, and he may not even know or care much about what is in it.

too fast—you need the right foods and supplements to put up the strongest possible defense against the disease of aging, to which you would otherwise fall victim.

Our Immortality Edge supplement system is not huge or difficult; the first stage includes only five supplements, and in the second stage, after six weeks, we'll have you add a few more. We don't like popping a lot of pills, and we suspect that you don't, either. The trick is to take the ones that matter, which isn't easy, because there are thousands of them on the market, packaged in many different forms and dosages.

Stage One

The supplements we want you to take in stage one are omega-3 in the form of pharmaceutical-grade fish oil, acetyl-L-carnitine (ALCAR), berry-derived anthocyanidins, and N-acetylcysteine (NAC), which is a precursor to intercellular glutathione. (We will explain all these terms shortly.) In addition, we strongly recommend that you take a super-multivitamin that includes higher concentrations of the usual antioxidants, plus folic acid; magnesium; potassium; vitamins C, D, and E; and superfoods such as a green tea and broccoli extract.

The chart on this page includes our recommended dosages.

The Immortality Edge Supplement System: Stage One[a]

Supplement	Optimal Daily Nutritional Allowance[b]	When to Take
Omega-3 fish oil (DHA and EPA)	6 g (6,000 mg)	3,000 mg twice daily with meals
Acetyl-L-carnitine (ALCAR)	2,000 mg	1,000 mg morning, 1,000 mg evening
Extracts standardized to contain anthocyanins	700–2,100 mg	700 mg with each meal

N-acetylcysteine (NAC)	1,200 mg	600 mg morning, 600 mg evening

ªSuper-multivitamin amounts vary, depending on the brand. Take as directed on the bottle.
ᵇOptimal nutritional allowance (ONA) is a different standard from the recommended daily allowance (RDA); the RDA is sometimes, though not always, less than the ONA. Maximum benefit is derived from the ONA. These dosages are for adults.

The rationale behind our list follows.

Omega-3 Fish Oil

The most important supplement you can take is omega-3 fish oil that contains both eicosapentaenoic acid (EPA) and docosahexaenoic acid (DHA). Ideally, fish oil should be taken with food once in the morning and once in the evening. During times of extraordinary stress or physical duress, such as joint pain, increase the dosage to 9,000 milligrams.

When we first considered fish oil as our number one Immortality Edge supplement, there weren't any specific data to suggest that fish oil was in any way linked to telomere length. We were on the verge of choosing it anyway, because it has so many phenomenal proven benefits backed up by literally thousands of independent scientific studies. Then, voilà, did we ever get lucky! A medical study in the *Journal of the American Medical Association (JAMA)* looked at how quickly telomeres shorten in people with coronary artery disease by following 608 participants for an average of five years, recording the amount of fish oil each consumed. Those with the greatest dietary intake of EPA and DHA fish oil had the longest telomeres. Those with the lowest consumption had the shortest telomeres.

Fish oil is known as an essential omega-3 fatty acid for the simple reason that your body cannot make it. It can come only from the outside—from your diet. As with all essential vitamins and minerals, there must also be a relatively constant intake, because it is burned up (oxidized) in everyday living. The more stress you are under, especially physical stress like exercise and dieting, the more you need to be aggressive about your fish oil.

Scientists love to use the word *pleomorphic* to describe the effects of fish oil. What they mean by this is that it is capable of taking many forms. It resides in many different places, where it performs different functions, as follows:

- *In the bloodstream.* Fish oil helps reduce inflammation in your body as it circulates through the bloodstream. Since blood goes everywhere in your body, fish oil's anti-inflammatory effects are far-reaching, and, as we all know, stopping inflammation is one of the keys to reversing age-related diseases.
- *In the cell membrane.* There are trillions of cells in our bodies, and every one of them contains some omega-3 fatty acids. It is particularly easy to detect the presence of omega-3 fatty acids in brain cells and red blood cells. Fish oil has been used to treat depression and other mood disorders as well as attention-deficit disorder, schizophrenia, and borderline personality disorder.
- *Inside the cell.* There is a whole emerging field of human biochemistry called *nutrigenomics*, which is the study of how food and supplements affect the human genetic code. Fish oil works at multiple levels of genetic expression, both in signaling and in transcription right at the level of the gene itself (DNA), where fish oil represses cancer-causing genes and helps to express healthier genes. There are studies that show it directly protects the DNA itself from oxidation, even though Western medicine does not consider it an antioxidant.

The evidence continues to mount that fish oil not only has innumerable anti-inflammatory, anticancer, and hypertensive effects, it is also crucial to the prevention and treatment of macular degeneration, arthritis, allergies, dementia, and Alzheimer's disease.

DHA is the most prominent fatty acid in the brain and is necessary for vision and cognitive function. Study after study has shown that the brains of Alzheimer's patients have a lower concentration of DHA than do the brains of individuals without this disease. The Rotterdam Study, conducted in 2003, found that ingesting fish oil once a week by eating fish or taking a supplement was associated with a 60 percent reduction in the risk of dementia.

Numerous findings on fish and fish oil report improved triglycerides, high-density lipoprotein (HDL) cholesterol (the "good" cholesterol), platelet function, endothelial (the lining of the blood vessels) and vascular function, blood pressure, cardiac excitability, measures of oxidative stress, reduced pro-inflammatory and increased anti-inflammatory cytokines (signaling molecules in the immune system), and enhanced immune function. Both EPA and DHA are constituents of the membranes of all cells in the body and precursors of locally produced eicosanoids. Eicosanoids derived from EPA and DHA help to reduce inflammation and promote health, while eicosanoids derived from omega-6 fatty acids promote inflammation. This is why it is very important to get plenty of omega-3 fatty acids and not too many omega-6 fatty acids in your diet.

No single drug or supplement has been as well researched and shown to have as many benefits. People who maintain consistently high levels of omega-3 fatty acids, like those found in fish oil, in their bodies have not only less cancer, less cardiovascular disease, less arthritis, and a significantly reduced risk of dementia but also a much lower risk of dying from any causes in the next ten years.

Fish Oil's Double Role in Telomerase

This may seem shocking, but laboratory studies show that fish oil effectively inhibits telomerase in cancer cells. This may explain why it is such an effective anticancer agent, but doesn't this also mean that fish oil suppresses telomerase in normal cells? If that were true, wouldn't the *JAMA* study cited previously have found the opposite results? Allow us to explain.

Fish oil is what scientists call an *adaptogen*, a substance that acts to bring some factor or measurement back to normal. Russian

scientists who were studying ginseng discovered this characteristic in the 1950s. They were astonished to find that if a person's
blood pressure was low, ginseng would help to raise it; conversely,
if the blood pressure was high, ginseng helped to lower it.

Side Effects

Fish oil is a fat (although it is often successfully used to decrease
body fat), so not everyone can tolerate bigger doses. If your gall-
bladder is missing and you have trouble digesting fatty foods,
you may have to take smaller doses for a while. Some people get
diarrhea on bigger doses, or burp. Burping of fish oil is often considered a sign that the supplement is of poor quality, and many
times it is. Rancid fish oil does you no good and may actually
harm you. Ask the manufacturer of your fish oil to provide a certificate of analysis indicating that the product is free of contami-
nants and has a low level of oxidation. If they cannot supply this
certificate, do not use their products.

Some people will always burp from fish oil, no matter what,
but storing it in the freezer and taking it with food may decrease
that effect. Most people find that as they take fish oil for longer
and longer, this side effect seems to disappear.

One potentially dangerous side effect with fish oil is blood
thinning. For most of us, this is a good thing, because we don't
have enough fish oil in our bodies to begin with. However, if
you are taking any drugs that thin the blood, including aspirin
and Coumadin (warfarin), caution should be used in combining them with fish oil. Recent studies have shown that although
there is no increase in bleeding with high doses of fish oil, any
medical condition in which anemia, bleeding, or easy bruising
is present is a reason to at least consult your doctor about fish
oil use.

A very small number of people are allergic to fish oil. If you
have a shellfish allergy, you can probably take fish oil if you consult
your doctor, but you should avoid shellfish-derived omega-3 fatty
acids, such as those from mussels and shrimplike organisms.

Why Can't I Just Eat Fish?

Just as with broccoli and blueberries, you could never eat enough fish to maintain the optimal levels of fish oil that we recommend—you'd have to wolf down six salmon fillets a day! In addition, one of the sadder facts of our modern world is that we've polluted our oceans and streams so badly that it is impossible to find fish that isn't contaminated with mercury and other toxins, including polyvinyl chloride (PVC) and polychlorinated biphenyls (PCBs), which cause cancer. The only way to guarantee that you are getting uncontaminated fish oil is to use a purified fish oil supplement that has been molecularly distilled.

As for fish oil substitutes, including plant-based substances like Salba (chia) and flaxseed or marine-based substances like krill or green mussels, we urge caution. Whereas fish oil has been tested for more than forty years in labs and human studies, including population-based studies, these other products have not. If you are a vegetarian or a vegan and just can't bring yourself to take fish oil, then algae-based omega-3 is probably the best source, but it's not as potent, and it is much more expensive on a per-milligram basis.

There is a common misperception that flaxseed or flax oil is an adequate substitute for fish oil. It is not. Fish oil contains the preformed omega-3 fatty acids EPA and DHA. Flaxseed oil, in contrast, contains the omega-3 fatty acid alpha-linolenic acid, which is the precursor of the omega-3 fatty acids in fish oil. The body can convert the alpha-linolenic acid in flaxseed oil to EPA and DHA, but the converted amounts seem to be minimal. Although flaxseed oil is thought to be heart-healthy in its own right, you can't count on it as a substitute for fish oil.

Krill is particularly suspect because it is eaten exclusively by whales, and whale meat is generally toxic to humans because of its high mercury content. If you must take krill, make sure it has been purified.

Other marine substitutes are possibly useful for people, but beware of marketing ploys such as "it's better than fish oil," "it's sustainable," or "it's green." Fish oil has been produced in a "green" fashion, with low carbon emissions, for a long time. In addition, it has been independently studied by unbiased institutions such as the American College of Cardiology, which recently changed its stance by recognizing fish oil as valuable for treating heart disease.

The bottom line is that there are two ways to increase your intake of fish oil omega-3 fatty acids: eat a whole lot of fish (risking mercury contamination) or take a high-quality fish oil supplement.

Acetyl-L-Carnitine

Acetyl-L-carnitine (ALCAR) is a modified form of the nutrient L-carnitine, which is naturally produced by the liver and the kidneys to help the body turn fat into energy. To modify, or acetylate, L-carnitine, an acetyl group (oxygen, carbon, and hydrogen atoms) is added to its molecular structure. This may sound esoteric, but it is a process common to several pharmaceuticals.

Used for years by athletes to perform longer at high-intensity levels and to recover more quickly after exercise, ALCAR plays a crucial role in energy production in the body. When your muscles have enough ALCAR, they can easily burn fat or protein (and not just glucose) for energy. This delays muscle fatigue, decreases the accumulation of lactic acid (a by-product of glucose metabolism), and spares glycogen, the stored form of glucose. ALCAR also increases the production of testosterone, which boosts muscle and bone mass, sex drive, and mood in both men and women.

The only documented side effect of ALCAR is diarrhea, and this occurs mostly at doses much, much higher than we recommend here.

ALCAR and the Brain

It's when ALCAR meets the brain, however, that things get really exciting.

One of the consequences of acetylating L-carnitine is that it becomes more effective at passing through the blood-brain barrier. Once that happens, it plays a role in the production of acetylcholine, a neurotransmitter that is vital to the proper functioning of the brain and the entire nervous system. A number of sound clinical studies have shown that ALCAR supplementation may help in reducing the mental decline due to aging, alcoholism, Alzheimer's disease, and reduced blood flow to the brain (chronic cerebral ischemia). Although your body can convert some L-carnitine to ALCAR, taking ALCAR itself is better for getting brain food.

More recent research indicates that ALCAR works in the brain through a group of genes called *vitagenes*. Vitagenes are very important; they protect our vital organ systems at the cellular level from oxidative stress, and they repair and strengthen mitochondria.

ALCAR and Mitochondria

Mitochondria are very tiny organelles (special cellular parts analogous to organs) that act like a digestive system inside cells. They take in nutrients, break them down, and create energy for the cell in a process called *cellular respiration*. Another way to look at mitochondria is to compare them to the internal combustion engine that runs an automobile. Just as the automobile engine creates a small amount of black smoke, the mitochondria create a small amount of free radicals; just as the engine emits more smoke as it gets older, the older the mitochondria get, the more free radicals they are likely to release.

According to Bruce Ames, a University of California, Berkeley, scientist who has researched mitochondria perhaps more than all other scientists combined, "Ten percent of mitochondria is eaten up every day. Your cells create new mitochondria but over time don't quite keep up." Every cell in the body has mitochondria. Brain cells, however, have more than a thousand. Although the brain is small in mass compared to the rest of the body, it uses a disproportionate amount of oxygen and energy to keep running.

If you get no oxygen in your body, your brain stops functioning faster than any other organ.

By repairing and strengthening mitochondria, ALCAR is indirectly doing something else of vital importance: it's protecting your telomeres. Just as car engines with dirty oil throw off black smoke, ailing mitochondria throw off free radicals. The more free radicals, the faster the wear and tear on the telomeres.

Berry-Derived Anthocyanidins

Anthocyanidins are the red-blue pigments that give many plants their color. They are flavonoids (antioxidant compounds), but unlike other flavonoids they are not bonded to sugar. The food sources of anthocyanidins are red and black grapes, red wine, bilberries, cranberries, strawberries, blueberries, red cabbage, and apple peel. Other sources include pine bark, grape seeds, bilberry leaves, birch, and ginkgo biloba.

Berries are the most underrated and underutilized source of potent antioxidants known to humanity. Containing particularly dense concentrations of anthocyanidins, berries and the extracts derived from them, including resveratrol, have been shown to promote cardiovascular health and to protect cells from the mutagenic (mutation-inducing) effects of cancer-causing nitrosamines (toxic food preservatives).

So we want you to take resveratrol, right? Actually, we don't, unless you take other antioxidants along with it. Despite the hype about resveratrol and all the press it is getting, there are few if any human studies that support its use. Scientists and entrepreneurs use the term *mammal studies* freely, but these most often refer to genetically modified mice, not people!

As for getting benefits from the resveratrol in red wine: sure, if your liver can tolerate drinking about a thousand glasses a day, go ahead!

If resveratrol isn't the answer, then blueberries are, correct? Nope, wrong again. Blueberries are great, and we all eat them as often as we can, but elderberries are actually more effective in combating both influenza A and B.

Employed as a remedy for centuries, elderberry juice is used for its antioxidant activity, to lower cholesterol, to improve vision, to boost the immune system, to improve heart health, and as protection from coughs, colds, flu, bacterial and viral infections, and even tonsillitis.

More recently it has been used to combat flu and flulike symptoms. In several large studies, people with the flu who drank elderberry juice reported less severe symptoms and felt better much faster than those who did not.

In addition to containing anthocyanidins, elderberries contain tannin, amino acids, carotenoids, other flavonoids, sugar, rutin, viburnic acid, vitamins A and B, and a large amount of vitamin C. In Israel, Hadassah Hospital's oncology lab has determined that elderberry stimulates the body's immune system, and the lab is treating cancer and AIDS patients with it. The wide range of medical benefits is probably due to this factor: strengthen the immune system, and all sorts of good things happen.

At the Bundesforschungsanstalt research center in Karlsruhe, Germany, scientists who conducted studies on elderberries found that elderberry anthocyanidins boost the production of cytokines. These unique proteins act as messengers in the immune system to trigger inflammation and to regulate immune response, thus helping to defend the body from disease by mobilizing antiviral immune cells in a very specific manner. Further research indicated that the anthocyanidins found in elderberries possess appreciably more antioxidant capacity than either vitamin E or vitamin C.

Berry-derived anthocyanidins—in a similar fashion to ALCAR—seem to work with vitagenes, which probably explains the anthocyanidins' anticancer properties. You can benefit from eating the fruit or drinking elderberry juice, but by now you know what we have to say about that. You'd have to eat a bushel basket of berries every day to get the dosage we recommend

(800 milligrams daily of potent berry extracts standardized to contain anthocyanins and other polyphenols).

Extracts and liquids of these berries often have pretty high alcohol content and lots of added sugar, so be careful about using them. We strongly recommend that you take "ultra" or "flash" pasteurized capsulized extracts instead. Flash-pasteurized extracts like these are available on a limited basis from very few companies, in particular from our own Dr. Dave's Web site, www .drdavesbest.com.

N-Acetylcysteine

The acetylated form of the amino acid L-cysteine, N-acetylcysteine (NAC) is rapidly metabolized in the body, where it becomes a precursor to intercellular glutathione.

Increasing the body's level of glutathione, which is considered the master antioxidant, is the whole point. You can take glutathione as a supplement, but unless it is injected directly into the bloodstream, very little of it will pass through to the cells. This, of course, doesn't stop unscrupulous vitamin makers from marketing glutathione, but it does make it suspect as a valuable supplement.

A new form of glutathione, one that is rubbed on the body as a cream instead of being taken orally, is in the works as we write this book. If and when it becomes available, assuming that its efficacy is adequately demonstrated, we will recommend this. Meanwhile, NAC will do nicely.

Glutathione is used to detoxify the body and to help it repair the damage caused by stress, pollution, radiation, infection, drugs, poor diet, aging, injury, trauma, and burns. Studies using either intravenous glutathione or oral NAC have shown improved heart function, improved blood-sugar numbers in diabetics, and improved response to exercise, especially when combined with whey protein.

Because glutathione occurs within the body's cells, it not only neutralizes free radicals, as other antioxidants do, it also keeps the cells running smoothly. One extremely important way it does this is by improving the body's ability to remove and recycle sick, dying, and dead cells. Through a process called *autophagy*, the cells actually recycle a large number of protein components from broken-down tissues. As a result, the body doesn't have to constantly maintain huge protein stores and can go for at least a time without dying of starvation.

Autophagy is a delicate process. If the autophagy system is disrupted by too much or too little fasting, sleep disturbances, or sugar problems like those associated with diabetes or high-carbohydrate diets, your body will have a harder time protecting itself from toxic onslaughts in the environment, such as pesticides and other poisons in food. The sick and dying cells will pile up in your system and basically clog up the works. The result looks an awful lot like aging!

A poorly functioning autophagic system will undoubtedly place more demands on the body to replace the sick, dying, and dead cells. Theoretically, this means more cell replication, more cell turnover, and faster shortening of your telomeres. Remember, every time a cell divides, its telomeres shorten. Anything that accelerates your cell-replication process in the absence of a telomerase activator—to lengthen telomeres and try to keep pace with the natural shortening process—accelerates the loss of telomeres.

Like ALCAR, glutathione plays an important role in keeping mitochondria healthy. If mitochondria, as we mentioned previously, are the body's internal combustion engines, then glutathione is the oil for the engine.

The Super-Multivitamins

The super-multivitamins we have in mind may require that you take more than one capsule. Some multivitamins can be taken once a day with a meal, whereas others have to be spread out over two or three meals.

High-quality super-multivitamins provide a rich and nearly complete list of vitamins, minerals, and other nutrients. This is one area in your life where you shouldn't skimp—don't buy the cheap multivitamins that are sold in the drugstore (with names like Dr. Joe's One-a-Day). Splurge on yourself and buy the best you can find.

A super-multivitamin includes, at minimum, the following supplements in the following amounts:

Super-Multivitamins*

Multivitamin Ingredient	Minimum Amount
Vitamin C	3,000 mg
Vitamin E	400 IU
Vitamin D	2,000 IU
Vitamin A	2,000 IU
Thiamine (vitamin B$_1$)	100 mg
Riboflavin (vitamin B$_2$)	100 mg
Niacin (vitamin B$_3$)	100 mg
Vitamin B$_6$	100 mg
Folic acid	800 mcg
Vitamin B$_{12}$	250 mcg
Biotin	100 mcg
Pantothenic acid	100 mg
Calcium	100 mg
Iodine	75 mcg
Magnesium	200 mg
Zinc	10 mg
Selenium	100 mcg
Potassium	10 mg

Choline	25 mg
Citrus bioflavonoids	50 mg
Broccoli concentrate	200 mg
Green tea extract	50 mg
Ginger root extract	25 mg
Cocoa	25 mg
Milk thistle extract	50 mg
Lutein	10 mg
Lycopene	2 mg
Grape seed	10 mg

*If you need help finding a super-multi that fits these requirements, see the list we have provided in the resources section at the end of this book.

Hundreds of studies have shown the benefits of multivitamins, covering the gamut of age-related diseases and even proving beyond a reasonable doubt that those who take multivitamins live substantially longer than those who don't. The study, however, that really matters to us and to *The Immortality Edge* was published in the *American Journal of Clinical Nutrition* in June 2009. Researchers from the National Institute of Environmental Health Sciences, led by Dr. Honglei Chen, looked at the length of telomeres. Dr. Chen and his coworkers analyzed the multivitamin use, nutrient intake, and telomere length of 586 women between the ages of thirty-five and seventy-four. A 146-item food-frequency questionnaire was used to determine multivitamin use and nutrient intake. Compared to people who did not take a multivitamin, the people who took a multivitamin daily had telomeres that were, on average, 5.1 percent longer.

In an attempt to identify the specific nutrients that could be behind these observations, the researchers observed a positive relationship between telomere length and the intake of vitamins C and E from food.

This study provides the first epidemiological evidence that multivitamin and micronutrient use is associated with longer telomere length, and others will surely follow. Meanwhile, if you aren't already taking vitamins, start popping those pills!

There are other good supplements as well. Once you've gotten used to taking the ones we have recommended here—you tolerate them well and are in the habit of consistently taking them with a meal every day—it will be time to up the ante with a few additional supplements.

Stage Two

You're eating the right foods and have been taking the basic supplements for about six weeks. Now it's time to do more. There are five other supplements we recommend for optimal cellular health and telomere protection. Think of it this way: if the pills you are taking as a result of following our recommendations in stage one represent a tasty "health cake," then the ones below are the icing on the cake. In addition, you'll have the option of taking the one and only supplement that has been proven to actually lengthen telemeres and not just slow down their shortening. This is the cherry on top.

We realize that the supplement list is getting rather long, but it will pay off in the long run, and you may discover some immediate benefits from adding them to your routine. One way to find out if you can feel a difference is to take the sets of supplements in two stages, as we recommend.

The two-stage approach makes sense if you want to measure the markers of inflammation in your blood, because you can have a before-and-after comparison. Have a blood test before you start on stage one, have another before you start on stage two, and then have a third one six weeks to two months after you have been on the complete program.

Be proactive with your doctor; tell (don't just ask) him or her that you want to measure your C-reactive protein and homocysteine levels, because these are the two most common and easy ways to measure inflammation.

The first, C-reactive protein (CRP), is a substance made by your liver and secreted into the bloodstream, and it increases when inflammation is present. It is a sensitive marker of systemic (affecting your entire body) inflammation, which has emerged as a powerful predictor of coronary heart disease and other diseases of the cardiovascular system. Systemic inflammation is also linked with the onset of type 2 diabetes, age-related macular degeneration, the loss of cognitive skills, and rheumatoid arthritis. A CRP reading of lower than 3 milligrams per deciliter is considered optimal, whereas higher levels may indicate serious underlying inflammatory problems.

Increased concentrations of the second marker, homocysteine, have been associated with an increased tendency to form unwanted blood clots. The optimal level of homocysteine for both men and women is lower than 7 to 8 micromoles per liter.

Be aware that these tests are not always included in the typical blood test taken during a physical exam, and you might even have to pay for them, depending on your health insurer. If you want to avoid the hassle and extra expense of being tested through your doctor, you can order the tests yourself online through a number of services. One site that we recommend is www.LifeExtension.com/blood, because they use a nationwide network of reputable labs, including LabCorp, and they also provide free access to health advisors to assist you in understanding what your results mean.

After following our supplement plan, you should see definite improvements in the follow-up tests for both CRP and homocysteine. If not, definitely see your doctor. Also, keep in mind that it's a good idea to take all of your supplements with meals so that your body treats them as food. After all, they are food supplements!

Now let's look at the supplements you should add in stage two.

The Immortality Edge Supplement System: Stage Two

Supplement[a]	Optimal Daily Nutritional Allowance[b]
Coenzyme Q_{10} (CoQ_{10})	200 to 600 mg
L-carnosine[c]	1,000 mg to a maximum of 5,000 mg
Phosphatidylserine (PS)	100 to 800 mg
Alpha-lipoic acid (ALA)	50 to 300 mg
Vitamin D	2,000 to 10,000 IU

[a]All of these can be taken with any meal.
[b]Optimal nutritional allowance (ONA) is a different standard from the recommended daily allowance (RDA); the RDA is sometimes, though not always, less than the ONA. Maximum benefit is derived from the ONA. These dosages are for adults.
[c]Not to be confused with acetyl-L-carnitine.

Why Is CoQ_{10} So Important?

Coenzyme Q_{10} (ubiquinone), or CoQ_{10}, is a potent antioxidant that helps the mitochondria, the powerhouses in your cells, to stay young, which results in greater vitality for your cells and your telomeres. We noted earlier that mitochondria are like the engine in your car. They burn fuel and air to make power, thereby providing us with more than 98 percent of the energy we need to live. Mitochondria are walled off from the rest of the cell by two special membranes whose function is to protect the sensitive proteins and the genetic material that are stored and used outside the mitochondria from the stuff inside, which is highly toxic to the rest of the cell. It's like having a nuclear power plant in your basement.

Vital organs, including the heart, the brain, the pancreas, and the liver, have a higher concentration of mitochondria than other tissues do. As we age, our mitochondria start to lose their efficacy in generating power. Like an old engine, they no longer burn fuel cleanly; instead they start to produce gunk or, to continue the car metaphor, "black smoke" that clogs up our bodies and affects just about every other cellular process. Our power output declines and we start to form more and more free radicals.

In recent years, researchers have discovered that the decline in mitochondrial strength and numbers mirrors the concentration of CoQ_{10}. The more CoQ_{10}, the more mitochondria.

What is the connection to the telomere, the key to cell aging? This bears repeating: the telomere is truly a biological clock, because it controls whether the cell replicates. When the cell is exposed to low-level or moderate-level stresses, it shortens the telomere faster than normal. This means that the cell ages faster. Telomere length is really the on-off switch for several processes that cause the cell to "stall," in effect, and stop replicating. If you start damaging the telomere faster than normal, it will stall sooner. If you damage it at a higher level, it will actually tell the cell to commit suicide! This means that when the mitochondria lose their ability to buffer the free radicals and instead release more of them into the cell, the pace of telomere shortening quickens.

Telomeres are located only in our chromosomes, which are located in the nuclei of the cells that are separated from the mitochondria. What's important here is that telomeres ultimately depend on energy for their maintenance and upkeep.

CoQ_{10} helps to keep up the energy output inside the cells so they can do self-maintenance and thereby keep our genetic material, including our telomeres, healthy. CoQ_{10} protects telomeres by slowing shortening. (Some studies that used various forms of CoQ_{10} suggest that it can actually stop shortening altogether.) This makes CoQ_{10} a key component of your supplement routine.

Why, then, have we relegated CoQ_{10} to the second stage—the "frosting"? If it's so helpful, why isn't it part of the "cake"? It's mainly a matter of cost. CoQ_{10} is among the more expensive supplements. When you shop for it, you'll find it packaged in dosages from 30 to 400 milligrams. A month's supply of the 200 milligram version runs about fifty dollars. If you take 400 milligrams per day, it will cost you twice this. It's expensive, but it's cheaper than health insurance and arguably better.

We do not recommend the ubiquinone forms of CoQ_{10}. They are far less expensive but are poorly absorbed and have never been studied for their effect on telomeres. Instead, use softgels containing ubiquinol, which has been shown in studies to be much more absorbable.

L-Carnosine

The next supplement we recommend as part of an anti-aging, telomere-saving routine is L-carnosine (not to be confused with L-carnitine or acetyl-L-carnitine). A combination of two important amino acids, beta-R-alanine and histidine, it occurs naturally in humans and is highly concentrated in our muscles, hearts, and brains.

L-carnosine can be easily broken down into its two components, but these amino acids work much more efficiently if taken together. They are a powerful duo that rejuvenates cells, so we can stay with L-carnosine and avoid beta-R-alanine. For years, bodybuilders and other athletes have sworn by L-carnosine for reducing fatigue during workouts and for boosting energy. From hundreds of studies we know that L-carnosine possesses strong antioxidant properties that protect us from radiation damage, improve heart function, promote quicker recovery from injuries, and play important roles as a neurotransmitter, a modulator of enzyme activities, and a chelator of heavy metals, including lead, arsenic, and mercury.

The list of benefits goes on. The evidence suggests that L-carnosine may also boost immunity, reduce inflammation, prevent the formation of gastric ulcers, help to eradicate *Helicobacter pylori* (which are linked to peptic ulcers and stomach cancer), reduce the formation of beta-amyloids (which are found in the brains of people with Alzheimer's disease), prevent cataract formation, and reduce the effects of glucose damage and protein oxidation.

Until recently, scientists had no clue why L-carnosine has such a large number of beneficial properties. Thanks to research at the Chinese Academy of Sciences in Beijing, however, we now have a strong indication that L-carnosine dramatically reduces the rate of telomere shortening. The Beijing scientists studied the rate of growth and the life spans of human fetal lung connective tissue (fibroblast) cells in concentrations of L-carnosine and compared this to cells grown without these concentrations. The cells grown in L-carnosine exhibited slower telomere shortening, and their life spans doubled. Subsequent studies suggest that L-carnosine also increases the number of cellular replications and may actually be a telomerase activator.

If you don't take this supplement, your body will still get the L-carnosine it needs if you eat red meat, poultry, and fish. If you're a vegetarian, you're surely deficient and really need to take L-carnosine as a supplement. If you are not a vegetarian, you may or may not be getting enough, depending upon how much animal flesh you're consuming on a regular basis. What exactly is enough? To have an impact on cellular aging and thus your telomeres, plus all the other benefits above, you need an optimal L-carnosine level in your system, not just the recommended daily allowance. This is why we recommend 500 milligrams for both vegetarians and omnivores.

Phosphatidylserine

The next item in our anti-aging arsenal is phosphatidylserine (PS). A member of a class of lipids (fats) known as phospholipids, PS is an essential component of our cell membranes. A type of skin that surrounds the cells, cell membranes not only keep the cells intact, they also perform important functions that include moving nutrients into the cells and pumping waste out of the cells.

When deficient in PS, cell membranes aren't as porous as they should be, and, metaphorically speaking, our cells simultaneously starve and become constipated. Low-fat and low-cholesterol diets lack up to 150 milligrams per day of dietary PS, and a vegetarian diet may undersupply as much as 200 milligrams per day. Diets low in omega-3 fatty acids may reduce the amount of PS in the brain by as much as 28 percent, thereby impairing its ability to form, store, process, and remember. This dietary shortage is compounded by aging, because as you age your brain needs more PS, and your digestive system is less efficient at producing it. Modern industrial production of fats and oils also tends to decrease natural phospholipids, including PS.

When our cell membranes contain an optimal amount of PS, all sorts of wonderful things happen. More than three thousand studies have shown that PS is highly effective in slowing memory loss, increasing thinking ability, and intensifying concentration power. In some parts of Europe it is even used to treat Alzheimer's disease. In the United States, it is marketed primarily as a brain booster for people of all ages. Whether it actually prevents dementia is not conclusive, but there is little doubt that it can delay its onset.

We like PS for these reasons, but we like it even more for its ability to reduce stress by mitigating the effects of the stress hormone cortisol. Bodybuilders are known to take daily doses of 800 milligrams of PS to reduce the breakdown of muscle tissue caused by the surge of cortisol that is released in an intensive workout. This allows sore muscles to recover faster, so the bodybuilders can work out more often and become larger more quickly.

Scientists recently discovered that PS binds, and thereby inactivates, the stress hormone cortisol. Released by the adrenal glands as the result of sudden shock or traumatic events, cortisol causes the fight-or-flight response that is familiar to all of us.

There is most definitely a telomere connection with PS. Studies by Elizabeth Blackburn and others have shown that stress, and particularly chronic stress, speeds up the shortening of telomeres.

It makes sense that if you block the effects of the hormones that shorten telomeres, you block telomere shortening. The National Institute of Environmental Health Sciences looked at stressed-out telomeres and found that shortened telomeres are linked to shortened life span and increased cancer risk. Moderate stress and even perceived stress correlated with shorter telomeres, as well. Also, the longer that stress continues, the more damage it does.

By helping our bodies deal with cortisol and stress, PS helps our cells to stay healthy, and this in turn extends the life span. What could be more logical?

Alpha-Lipoic Acid: An Antioxidant Champion

Like PS, alpha-lipoic acid (ALA) is a fat found inside every one of our cells. But it's not a phospholipid; it's a sulfur-containing fatty acid that is both fat- and water-soluble, which means that it can get into all cell parts, where it neutralizes free radicals. This is one of its key features—it goes where other antioxidants cannot.

Discovered in the 1950s, ALA has only recently become one of the most recognized and sought-after health supplements. This is because of its potency—it is up to four hundred times more powerful than vitamins C and E combined—and because it seems to work well in synergy with many of the other supplements.

One example is ALCAR, which we recommended to you earlier. Working together, ALA and ALCAR have been shown to increase the number of mitochondria, particularly in brain tissue, and by doing this, to provide extra energy, sharper and better memory, more restful sleep, healthier blood pressure, and even shinier hair and younger-looking skin.

This is not all. ALA increases your body's sensitivity to insulin, which in turn enhances its ability to build lean body mass and reduce fat. Like ALCAR, it combines well with another popular bodybuilding supplement, creatine, to provide an energy boost. (Unless you are a serious athlete, we don't recommend creatine.)

ALA seems to have a positive impact on many diseases, including HIV, type 2 diabetes, hyperglycemia, glaucoma, cataracts, heart disease, and even Alzheimer's disease. It also seems to help treat hepatitis and obesity. It is used to support the best cardiovascular and mental health, liver function, eye health, and a healthy immune system, and it has been shown to protect the integrity of organ cells, particularly in the brain and the liver.

The list goes on. ALA enhances the potency of glutathione, helps the liver to detoxify itself, and protects the brain from free-radical damage. A deficiency of ALA has been associated with strokes, dementia, Parkinson's disease, and Alzheimer's disease.

Your body produces ALA, but not enough to get the above benefits. Diet-derived ALA can prevent a deficiency, but it acts as an antioxidant only when there is an excess of it in a free state in your cells. Thus, you need to take it as a supplement. If you happen to be diabetic, you should discuss ALA with your doctor, because it has been known to reduce the need for diabetic medication, which means that your doctor might want to lower your meds first. Otherwise, the combination might cause your blood sugar number to drop too low, which could result in a whole host of unwanted problems.

Because the long-term effects of ALA are not known, we err on the side of a low dosage and suggest that you discuss this with your doctor before taking it. Because it works so well with other antioxidants, we think it is better to buy a comprehensive formula rather than the stand-alone version, preferably a combination with vitamins C and E or with ALCAR. Dr. Andrew Weil sells an ALA combination called Juvenon, which includes both ALCAR and biotin (a member of the vitamin B complex). Devised by the famous geneticist and biochemist Bruce Ames, Juvenon is marketed to aging baby boomers and others who want to effectively slow down the cellular aging process.

The specific effects of ALA on telomeres have not been adequately studied, so unlike the evidence for PS and some of the other supplements, there is no particular study that says it will stop telomere shortening or activate telomerase. The only remotely relevant study involved brain cells from rats and found that vitamin E enhanced with ALA did both, at least in vitro (in a test tube).

By now you understand the logic. Anything that increases energy and slows down cellular aging will, by definition, help telomeres to stay nice and long and healthy! Therefore, adding alpha-lipoic acid (ALA) to your supplement routine is a very good idea. We have a specific recommendation that you look for the R form of ALA as it is more potent, and especially the sodium salt form (see the vitamin chart on page 74).

Vitamin D₃: Hugely Important

As you probably know, vitamin D is called the *sunshine vitamin* because your body can manufacture it from sunlight. To appreciate the huge importance of this vitamin to your health, however, it is helpful to understand that, technically speaking, it is not really a vitamin. It's a hormone.

Vitamin D is a hormone that your body makes in assembly-line fashion. When sunlight strikes your skin, cholesterol turns the sunlight into a precursor of vitamin D, which circulates throughout the bloodstream. As it passes through your liver, it is turned into a biologically inactive 25-hydroxyvitamin D (this is what doctors measure to determine your vitamin D level). The kidneys then get into the action, supplying a small chemical adjustment that creates the active version of vitamin D. The active version of vitamin D is actually the hormone calcitriol, also known as vitamin D₃. Calcitriol is very powerful; it controls calcium and phosphorus absorption, bone metabolism, and neuromuscular function.

If you are not taking a vitamin D₃ supplement or drinking copious amounts of vitamin D–fortified milk (which does not fit our dietary recommendations) or orange juice, or eating lots of fish, the amount of 25-hydroxyvitamin D circulating in your body is dependent on how much sunshine you get, your skin pigmentation (darker skin means reduced vitamin D production), and your age. The older you are, the less vitamin D your skin makes.

People who live and work outdoors most of the day probably don't need to worry too much about vitamin D unless they use a sunscreen with a protection factor (SPF) of 8 or greater. Of course, season, latitude, time of day, cloud cover, and smog affect ultraviolet ray exposure. If you happen to live in Boston, for instance, the average amount of sunlight is insufficient to produce significant vitamin D synthesis in the skin from November through February, no matter how long you are outdoors. Unfortunately, the vast majority of adults in the United States and the industrialized world spend most daytime hours inside; consequently, millions of people are deficient in vitamin D.

Traditionally, vitamin D is associated with bone health, because it helps your digestive system to absorb calcium and phosphorus. Prior to the fortification of milk in the 1930s, the bone disease rickets was a major problem, particularly in children. Now it is uncommon. Today, vitamin D deficiency is still commonly associated with osteoporosis and hip fractures, but there is so very much more to this powerful vitamin—that is, hormone.

Dozens of new studies have found that vitamin D_3 affects human health in a much more profound way than was ever imagined. It is now well established that the active form of vitamin D acts as an effective regulator of cell growth and differentiation in a number of different cell types, including cancer cells. Vitamin D_3 most likely protects us from the four most common cancers: breast, prostate, colon, and skin.

A deficiency of Vitamin D_3 is a major factor in coronary artery disease, because the deposit of calcium in the arteries is more likely to happen in people who are deficient. This makes sense and is backed up by science. It is no surprise that a Harvard-based study found that men who were low in vitamin D were twice as likely to develop heart disease as those with plenty of the vitamin in their circulatory systems.

And there's more—a lot more. Vitamin D decreases the kidneys' production of renin, a hormone that boosts blood pressure. Low vitamin D thus contributes to high blood pressure, whereas getting more vitamin D can help to control it. Too little vitamin D can leave the body prone to infection, whereas having enough can help the body to fight off the flu, tuberculosis, and upper respiratory infections. A deficiency in vitamin D has also been linked to type 2 diabetes, depression, asthma, dementia, and many other chronic conditions.

What does this have to do with telomeres? Although there isn't yet direct evidence that vitamin D activates telomerase, there is some stunning evidence that it dramatically slows the rate of telomere shortening. A large study of female twins in England that compared telomere length with concentrations of vitamin D found that women with higher levels of vitamin D had longer telomeres. The difference between those with the highest concentrations and those with the lowest was the equivalent of five years of telomere aging. The researchers speculated that the reason is that vitamin D is a powerful inhibitor of inflammation and thereby reduces the stress on cells, keeping the telomeres from shortening too rapidly.

You might be wondering why we are talking about vitamin D here when we already included it in the super-multivitamins of stage one. The reason is that we think everyone should get his or her vitamin D levels measured by a doctor. There is always a chance that your levels are so low that you will need to take daily doses of 5,000 to 10,000 international units, or even higher, of vitamin D.

The latest scientific findings suggest that an ideal dose of vitamin D_3 is 2,000 to 5,000 international units daily, depending on your blood level of 25-hydroxyvitamin D. In order to enjoy optimal health, you should strive for a vitamin D blood level of 50 to 80 nanograms per milliliter.

We strongly recommend that the form of vitamin D you take is D_3. As a supplement, vitamin D is available in two distinct forms: D_2 (ergocalciferol) and D_3 (cholecalciferol). Until recently, nutritionists had considered the two forms equivalent and inter-changeable, but this perception was based on studies of rickets prevention in infants from seventy years ago. More recent studies have found D_3 to be nearly three times as potent as D_2 in raising 25-hydroxyvitamin D levels in humans.

TA-65, for Those Who Want to Do It All

TA-65, a nutritional supplement available through doctors licensed by T. A. Sciences, has huge potential to extend your life; that's the good news. The bad news is that it currently costs from twenty-two hundred to eight thousand dollars per year, depending on the dosage. There's good news, though, that will make this supplement much less costly, without losing its effec-tiveness. We spoke to Noel Thomas Patton, founder of T. A. Sciences, as we were going to print, and he told us, "Long before *The Immortality Edge* is published we will have the peer-reviewed paper published by Dr. Calvin Harley that clearly demonstrates TA-65's effectiveness at lower doses than that which costs eight thousand dollars a year."

The lower doses, one that costs half of the current recom-mendation ($4,400 a year) and one that is one-quarter of the high price–tagged dose ($2,200 a year) are geared toward younger people (those who are just hitting their forties) and those whose budget precludes taking the more costly dose.

It may seem strange to put a price tag on your life, but we all do it every day without thinking about it. Every time we make a decision that affects our health and well-being based on what we can afford rather than what is best for us, we are putting a price tag on our lives. Before you object, consider how much money you spend on entertainment, vacations, eating out, and the like. For some people, this is clearly in excess of $2,400 to $8,000 dollars a year.

Keep that in mind as we describe the one and only proven telomerase activator that is available right now, in today's world: TA-65.

The TA-65 story begins in 2001. Hunting for a drug to treat chronic degenerative disease, Geron, then a small biopharmaceutical company in Menlo Park, California, began screening natural supplements that might target telomeres. After much trial and error, the Geron scientists discovered a single molecule in the astragalus plant (an ancient Chinese herbal medicine) that activates telomerase without any known toxicity. Because the company was more interested in finding ways to suppress telomerase in cancer cells, it licensed the rights to this molecule to a startup in New York City, T. A. Sciences, Inc.

Beginning in 2002, T. A. Sciences spent five years testing and developing a highly concentrated form of astragalus, which it called TA-65. In 2005, the company was able to demonstrate through a double-blind, placebo-controlled study that people who took TA-65 showed marked improvement in measurable anti-aging biomarkers. Specifically, their immune systems were strengthened, some showed vision improvement, many showed increased sexual function, others reported that their energy levels rose, and skin elasticity improved for some (that is, they had younger-looking skin).

Even more exciting is that in 2007, an independent company, Sierra Sciences in Reno, Nevada, was able to prove that TA-65 does indeed activate telomerase. Later studies conducted in Spain proved that TA-65 caused critically short telomeres to lengthen.

Because it is marketed as a supplement, TA-65 needs no approval from the FDA. One implication of this is that T. A. Sciences cannot make any claims about TA-65's ability to prevent or cure diseases, even though there is a provable link between telomere length and age-related disease. TA-65 has been commercially available since 2007 without any reported adverse effects. Nevertheless, the following questions remain about this supplement:

- Does it cause cancer?
- Will it come down in price? (We've already answered that one—yes!)
- Has the government or any major university tested it?

The question of cancer is frequently asked because telomerase is activated to a high degree in about 85 percent of human cancers. Thus it is a natural concern that something that seems to mimic what cancer does might cause cancer. Although it is not 100 percent proven, it appears that the way that TA-65 activates telomerase is mild and far more natural than the huge and multiple ways that it is activated in cancer. That is, TA-65 is closer to the natural telomerase activation that appears in stem-cell and germ-cell lines than to the unbridled and ungoverned ways that telomerase is turned on in cancer. To date, there are no studies linking TA-65 use to cancer in any way. In fact, given the proven immune function benefits there are those who speculate that TA-65 provides more "good guys to fight off the bad guys."

The price tag is not likely to come down again anytime soon, because the proprietary process of extracting one specific molecule from the astragalus plant is complicated, and the molecule is only one of more than two thousand found in the plant. There are other astragalus-based supplements on the market that claim to activate telomerase, but tests have proven that they don't. These are much cheaper because they contain no TA-65 and because they don't actually activate telomerase.

Sierra Sciences, as we noted in chapter 1, has screened about 250,000 compounds and found 770 inducers. None of these is powerful enough to be used as a drug, but the search goes on. Assuming that Sierra Sciences is successful in finding the right compound, it will then take the company many years to go through all the stages of developing, testing, and marketing an FDA-approved drug. Current choices are therefore limited.

If you want to take a pill that will absolutely turn on telomerase, improve immune function, and has been shown to lengthen critically short telomeres, TA-65 is the only option for now. You can learn more about TA-65 and find a list of doctors who are licensed to prescribe it at the T. A. Sciences Web site, www.tasciences .com, or by visiting www.telonauts.com, a Web site devoted to fans and followers of the technology and featuring some of the leading scientists in the field.

Additional Longevity Supplements

For readers who want to go beyond the two-stage program we have recommended here, we offer a complete list of longevity-related supplements below, with their optimal nutritional allowances and notes about their benefits.

The Immortality Edge Supplement System: Additional Supplements

Supplement	Primary Benefit(s)	ONA[a]	Notes
Acetyl-L-carnitine (ALCAR)[b]	Refreshes mental energy, improves mood, and slows the aging of cells—particularly brain cells. May impede the development of Alzheimer's disease.	500 to 1,000 mg twice daily	Best taken in combination with ALA.
Alpha-lipoic acid (ALA) (We recommend LifeExtension's Super R-Lipoic Acid.)	A powerful antioxidant that is readily absorbed into the body. Helps to control inflammation and repair collagen damage, which is why it is often found in antioxidant skin creams.	100 to 200 mg twice daily; 300 mg daily if you are using Super R-Lipoic Acid	When combined with ALCAR, it has been shown to repair mitochondria.
Berry-derived anthocyanidins[b]	A rich source of flavonoids; a wild berry extract, particularly chokecherry and black cherry. Effective in battling the type of inflammation that shortens telomeres.	700 mg daily	During times of stress or illness, double the dosage.
CoQ$_{10}$[b] as ubiquinol	Reduces the symptoms of heart disease, including congestive heart failure, and can aid in restoring the heart to its healthy state.	100 to 600 mg daily	People with heart disease should take 100 mg twice daily—400 mg of the ubiquinol form of CoQ$_{10}$.

Curcumin	A powerful anti-inflammatory agent derived from turmeric that provides protection from the multitude of mutagens in the environment. May be helpful in combating arthritis.	400 mg daily	People in India have been using this for centuries.
Vitamin D	Is associated with decreased risk of many common cancers, including colon, breast, prostate, and ovarian. Critical for maintaining calcium in the blood.	2,000 to 5,000 IU or more daily (Make sure your doctor follows your 25-hydroxyvitamin D level and adjusts your dose as needed. The optimum level ranges between 55 and 100 ng/ml.)	20 minutes a day of direct sunlight will provide a similar amount of vitamin D.
DHEA	A natural hormone that decreases with age. Increasing DHEA improves sex drive, enhances immunity, sharpens memory, and brightens mood.	25 to 50 mg daily (Your dose should be adjusted as needed based on a blood test called DHEA-S.)	Because DHEA can stimulate testosterone production, it should not be taken by men at risk for prostate cancer.
Vitamin E	Improves blood viscosity, protects the heart, and may help to reduce the risk of dementia. Combined with selenium, it can provide protection from methylmercury, the mercury contaminant detected in fish and seafood.	400 IU daily	Use natural, mixed tocopherols, not alpha-tocopherol.

(continued)

The Immortality Edge Supplement System: Additional Supplements (*Continued*)

Supplement	Primary Benefit(s)	ONA[a]	Notes
Vitamin K$_2$	Is essential for the formation of osteocalcin, the structural framework inside bones around which calcium crystallizes.	1,000 mcg once to three times daily	Warning: Vitamin K can counteract prescription anticoagulant such as warfarin. Consult your doctor.
L-carnosine[b]	Rejuvenates cells, reduces fatigue, counteracts inflammation, and reduces telomere shortening.	1,000 mg daily	May be a telomerase activator (not proven).
Lutein with zeaxanthin	Wards off cataracts, reduces the risk of macular degeneration, and reduces the fatigue caused by staring for long periods at a computer screen.	20 mg lutein and up to 8 mg zeaxanthin daily	These are the dominant carotenoids that protect the eyes. They are concentrated in kale, spinach, and other leafy greens, but few people eat enough of these.
Lycopene	A powerful carotenoid that reduces the risk of cancer.	15 mg daily	Tomato paste is one of the best natural sources of lycopene.
Magnesium	Reduces the risk of metabolic syndrome, including components such as high blood pressure, high blood sugar levels, elevated fats, and low levels of HDL cholesterol.	400 mg	Many medications, including diuretics, deplete the body of magnesium.

Melatonin	A natural hormone that induces sleep, fights sleep deprivation, and helps reduce jet lag.	1 to 10 mg nightly	The dosage varies because melatonin is more effective in some people than in others, and it is harmless to take up to 10 mg.
Milk thistle	Provides liver support, has been shown to reduce death from cirrhosis, and improves the outcome of hepatitis treatments.	150 to 600 mg daily in 2 to 3 divided doses	May offer liver protection from alcohol and other liver damage and help if your albumin levels are elevated.
Multivitamin[b]	Take one of the six brands recommended in the resources that includes the antioxidants selenium and vitamins C and E, plus superfoods green tea and broccoli.	Manufacturer's suggested dose	Make sure the supplement does not contain iron; this mineral can generate excess free radicals in those who are not deficient in it.
N-acetyl-cysteine (NAC)	Boosts gluthathione levels, supports detoxification, and helps maintain the integrity of cells and telomeres.	600 mg twice daily	It is normal for NAC to have a foul odor; it contains sulfur.
Omega-3 fish oil (DHA and EPA)	Promotes cardiovascular health and prevents heart attacks by lowering blood pressure and maintaining arterial flexibility. Reduces triglycerides and increases levels of HIDL cholesterol. Has been shown to lubricate joints and alleviate the symptoms of arthritis. May reduce the risk of Alzheimer's disease.	3,000 mg once to twice daily	

(continued)

The Immortality Edge Supplement System: Additional Supplements (*Continued*)

Supplement	Primary Benefit(s)	ONA[a]	Notes
Phosphatidylserine (PS)[b]	Stimulates the cells of the brain to make more dendrites and axons and thereby enhances cognitive function.	300 mg daily	People who take PS remember more names, faces, phone numbers, and other details.
Probiotics	Assist digestion and the absorption of fats and carbohydrates, fight bacterial infections, boost immunity, and may even promote longevity.	30 to 60 billion CFU daily, which is typically 1 to 3 pills	These are the "good" bacteria found in unpasteurized yogurt. However, it is impossible to get enough from yogurt alone.
Saw palmetto	Relieves constricted urinary flow by blocking the enzyme that causes the prostate to enlarge. Some men who take this also report sexual rejuvenation.	370 mg daily, standardized to 85 to 95 percent sterols and total fatty acids	Men only.
Selenium as methylselenocystein	A powerful antioxidant with proven cancer-fighting properties that seem to be effective against all forms of cancer.	200 mcg daily	Best taken with vitamin E. See vitamin E above.

[a]Optimal nutritional allowance (ONA) is a different standard from the recommended daily allowance (RDA); the RDA is sometimes, though not always, less than the ONA. Maximum benefit is derived from the ONA. These dosages are for adults.
[b]Recommended for telomere stability and the oxidative stress that threatens this stability.

3

The Immortality
Edge Fitness Plan

The people who make commercials for Nike aren't stupid. They know that since ancient times humans have admired the athletic human form at its hard-bodied best. Since the original Greek Olympic games and the marble statues that memorialize them, the athletes who push beyond the usual limits of performance are the ones we admire the most. So when Nike's photographers shoot those modern-day athletic heroes in ideal light as their bodies reach for excellence, the marketers add a powerful message for the rest of us: just do it.

Although perfection might be beyond the reach of most mere mortals, they don't have the advantage of a program based on the latest findings in telomere biology. You may very well surprise yourself with how much really can be accomplished, using what we've learned from the front lines of telomere biology, the science of exercise physiology, and our own enthusiasm for being as fit as possible.

Of course, much more important than looking fabulous is staying alive and healthy longer. Study after study reinforces the idea that a long healthy life is accomplished best by those who become and stay fit. In fact, exercise is so important that a lack of exercise is so bad for us that it might possibly speed up the time of our death. A six-year study of more than six thousand men (average age fifty-nine) by researchers at Stanford University found that those with the lowest exercise capacity (brought about because they didn't exercise) were more than four times as likely to die at any given time than the men with the highest exercise capacity. Now those are statistics, but they are telling, nonetheless. This was true even among the subjects who had cardiovascular disease. Exercise capacity, or the lack thereof, outranked even smoking and a history of chronic disease as a predictor of death. Studies of women have yielded similar results.

Better yet are the findings of a team of scientists from King's College, London, who discovered a significant link between telomere length and exercise among 2,401 identical and nonidentical twins (mostly women). The researchers determined how much exercise participants had done during the previous year, the subjects' body mass index (BMI), their socioeconomic status, and whether they were smokers.

Independent of all these variables, the researchers found that the more the volunteers exercised, the longer their telomere length was in their white blood cells. To make sure that genetics didn't account for these findings, the scientists checked their results by looking at a smaller group of identical twins who shared the same genes but differed in their levels of exercise. The link was confirmed.

Here's the kicker, though. The study found that the people who exercised vigorously three hours a week were biologically nine years younger than the people who exercised less than fifteen minutes a week. Moderate exercise, defined as ninety minutes a week, provided a four-year advantage.

"It is not just walking around the block," said Professor Tim Spector, the genetic epidemiologist who led the study, in a telephone interview. "It is really working up a sweat."

Exercise is also linked to lower rates of colon, prostate, and breast cancer. Study after study has shown the beneficial effect of exercise in treating mild to moderate depression, and even more eye-opening are the studies showing that seniors who engage in exercise at least three times a week cut their risk of Alzheimer's by as much as 40 percent.

The Birth of the Couch Potato

Once upon a time, unless you were very rich, life was full of physical activity. Transportation consisted of your own two feet, or if you were lucky you rode a horse. Farming was the main occupation and required hard manual labor from dawn to dusk. Without modern so-called labor-saving devices, washing, cooking, cleaning, and shopping were all serious workouts. Wealthy folks who had the luxury of avoiding such exertions turned up their noses at those labors, getting their workouts at the occasional formal dance or fox hunt but considering sweat as déclassé as dirty hands.

The industrial revolution radically changed our occupations and lifestyles. Machines started doing the hard jobs, at work and at home, and when radio, television, movies, and computers came along to fill the extra free time, we were only too happy to take a seat and a load off our feet. So our couch-potato culture was born—a twentieth-century phenomenon that is proving to be one of the greatest public health threats of the modern age.

Being a couch potato can create a vicious cycle, since being sedentary leaves you short on energy and verve. A variety of excuses keeps you sitting down. I don't have time. The gym is too far away. Gee, the weather looks nasty. I don't have a

(continued)

(continued)

workout buddy. There are more important things to do. I'll make up for it tomorrow or sometime soon. Here's the most insidious: I'll never have a perfect body, so why bother?

Our couch-potato problem may not come from a collective decision to go to pot as much as from the famous all-or-nothing American attitude. Many people think that unless a workout is time consuming and lasts hours, it is worthless, so they do nothing instead.

Exercise, however, is like saving for retirement: It's far more important that you do a little regularly than that you try to break any records by doing a lot all at once. Despite what your gym teachers or coaches might have shouted from the side-lines, there's no failing grade for exercise other than failing to exercise at all. Short exercise sessions are just as beneficial as long ones, particularly if they are intense, like the ones we recommend.

Looking great is wonderful, and if you exercise consistently enough you will start looking better and better. Meanwhile, being healthy, having more energy, and knowing you're on the path to living a much longer, rewarding life will just have to do!

We've learned a lot in recent years about how to stay in shape in the most efficient way, and in this chapter we'll explain the phenomenal benefits you'll receive from learning how to exercise using the principles of interval training and of training your fast-twitch muscle fibers as well as your slower ones.

We'll be really specific and provide you with a detailed, cus-tomizable Immortality Edge exercise program that will keep your telomeres long, prevent the possibility that you'll ever be weak and frail, and (we hope) keep you around long enough to benefit from the medical breakthroughs that will let you live for as long as you want. Before we get to that, however, we need to lay a solid foundation, or you simply might not believe how beneficial our high-intensity, time-saving exercise program is. Worse, you might not be sufficiently motivated to follow our revolutionary exercise program. We want to get you jazzed up first.

What elite athletes have that many of us want is a combination of the following: functional explosive strength, fast-twitch muscle fibers, and low body fat with well-defined muscles. You don't have to devote yourself to three hours a day in the gym (in fact, this plan will probably reduce the amount of time you exercise). Like elite athletes, you can learn from research to train in a targeted way for specific results—a healthier body that can live longer. And you can do it with far less discipline and effort than you might think.

Preparing for Exercise

Before you start any new exercise program, be sure you've seen your primary-care physician and gotten the essentials checked out. This will differ for people by age and gender, but a basic physical that measures your organ function and explores any chronic ailments or lingering pains is a good idea. You don't want to invite an injury by overdoing it with a body part that has been underused or has an underlying weakness, such as an arthritic joint.

Next, start out slowly. Get up to a decent level of fitness before you push really hard. This means that if you've been too busy to do your favorite cardio workout for the past few months, get going again, even if it is at a reduced rate. The same goes for resistance training—get out the weights or Pilates bands. Do whatever works for you.

Now you're ready to learn why shorter and faster exercise is actually better than long and repetitive exercise.

The Science of Exercise

Aging, in our view, is a battle between decay and growth. To stay young, you need to build up your body faster than it is being torn down. Exercise done properly is the best way to counteract the so-called aging process. Each time a person works out, his or her muscles should get stronger; enzymes and proteins flood the bloodstream, creating a controlled inflammation that triggers the repair process, which in turn triggers growth. The heart becomes stronger, more blood flows to the brain, the blood vessels become more flexible, the organs get more nourishment, and, most important, the immune system is invigorated. The trick, then, is to do a form of exercise that results in the least damage followed by the maximum growth.

In designing our fitness program, we looked for exercise that would absolutely provide the most fitness with the least damage. The fitness program we decided was best is derived from a tried and tested form of interval training called "Ready, Set, Go! Synergy Fitness," which was created by one of our expert advisers, Phil Campbell, a world-famous athlete and fitness trainer who started writing fitness manuals and managing health clubs more than thirty years ago. This exercise program involves a mixture of high-intensity bursts of exercise with moderate-intensity active recovery periods. Not only does our program produce the best results in the shortest time (twenty minutes), it also accomplishes this with the least bodily stress—and the least telomere shortening.

Next time you see one of those Nike ads featuring the stars of track and field, pay attention to how different the sprinters look from the marathoners. The sprinters have more developed muscles than the lean-bodied people who are running for hours at a time. It turns out that short bursts of high-intensity exercise build muscle. The human body is designed to create new muscle fibers that can meet the demands of speed and explosive movement. These muscle fibers are known as *fast-twitch* fibers. There are slow-twitch fibers as well, and they are developed by endurance exercise such as long-distance running.

Muscle Fibers

Let's take a minute to see what is happening in our muscles and cells as a result of the Immortality Edge program.

Muscle fibers come in a couple of different types. Slow-twitch muscle fibers burn fat and oxygen and fuel our activities throughout the day. This is what most recreational athletes use when they work out or play.

Fast-twitch explosive fibers burn primarily sugar and store short-term energy sources such as creatine. They burn almost no fat (although the work they do is a major stimulus for burning fat in the recovery phase). They kick in when you need explosive, fast, or very powerful, rapid reactions. Our Paleolithic ancestors had to run to save their lives from attack by saber-toothed tigers. Today, any New Yorker will tell you that it doesn't hurt to be able to race across a crosswalk in rush-hour traffic.

There is also an intermediate group, strength-endurance fibers, that covers the gray zone between fast- and slow-twitch fibers; they use both sugar and fat for fuel. These fibers allow us to crank up the exercise effort to somewhere between comfortable and maximum and sustain it for a while. These are the fibers that let those of us who are not genetically gifted with a lot of fast-twitch fibers to still win our local 10k race.

An ideal training program would give all three of these muscle fibers a workout and challenge all three to grow. This is the beauty of the workouts in the Immortality Edge program, which bypass time-wasting workouts and use all three fiber types.

The reason for this is very simple: When your workout is focused on slow-twitch fibers, they are the only ones that

(continued)

(continued)

benefit. Conversely, when your workout is focused on fast-twitch fibers, your body responds by trying to ramp up its ability to get both the slow-twitch and the strength-endurance fibers to do more of the work. Your body hates the maximum-intensity stuff, because it requires extra energy, so it looks for as much support as possible from the other fibers.

Pretty neat, huh?

One of the most valuable features of interval training is that it appeals to a broad spectrum of people: all ages and with an interest in many different kinds of exercise. Interval training can be readily adapted to swimming, running, biking, hiking, skiing, and even walking. You can also use the program on all kinds of gym equipment: a treadmill, a rowing machine, an elliptical trainer, or a spinning bike. You can even apply it to weight lifting. Chapter 7 includes an extensive chart that provides the reader with a large number of exercise choices at various levels of intensity.

Interval training is both aerobic and anaerobic. Most people are familiar with the former but not the latter. *Anaerobic*, which means "without oxygen," is a form of metabolism that relies on the energy that is stored in muscles (glycogen) for short, intensive bursts of activity. The by-product is lactic acid, which causes the burning sensation you feel in your muscles during high-intensity efforts. During high-intensity intervals, lactic acid builds up, and you enter what is called *oxygen debt*. During the recovery phase, the heart and the lungs work together to pay back this oxygen debt and break down the lactic acid. In this phase the aerobic system is in control, using oxygen to convert stored carbohydrates into energy.

This repetitive form of exercise leads to an adaptive response. The body begins to build new capillaries, and it is better able to take in and deliver oxygen to the muscles. The muscles, in turn, develop a higher tolerance to the buildup of lactate, and the heart muscle is strengthened. These changes result in improved performance, particularly within the cardiovascular system. Furthermore, all this is accomplished with minimal damage to the telomeres.

Just ask any high school or college athletes, whether they play basketball, football, soccer, or almost any other sport, which part of their daily practice they hate the most; nine times out of ten, the answer will be "wind sprints." Good coaches make their players run wind sprints to develop their breathing capacity during exertion and to push them past their comfort zone in order to develop maximum performance. And even though wind sprints are the shortest segment of a workout, in terms of strength, endurance, and speed they are the most beneficial.

Thus, by working out in shorter but harder segments, you actually kill three birds (three muscle-fiber types) with one stone. The net result is that you work out all of your muscle types, and your ability to do any and every type of workout improves.

Another thing that happens during this kind of quick-burst exercise is the release of human growth hormone (HGH), an important substance for keeping your cells young and happily burning fat. More muscle means less fat. You don't need a PhD in exercise physiology to know that that's a good thing. And as you might guess, growth hormone's role in cellular health is good for longevity.

While still controversial, countless studies show that HGH may reverse the signs of aging in at least a dozen measurable ways, including the following:

- Restoring muscle mass, lost hair, and the size of the liver, the heart, and other organs that shrink with age
- Decreasing body fat
- Increasing energy, sexual function, and cardiac output
- Improving cholesterol profile, vision, and memory
- Thickening skin and reducing wrinkles
- Normalizing blood pressure

Even more impressive, from our point of view, is some recent research in Italy that found that higher levels of HGH correlate with longer telomeres. Measurements for both were taken from 476 healthy people (both men and women) between the ages of 16 and 104, and after the effect of age was factored in, it was determined that high HGH levels accounted for a 10 percent increase in telomere length.

Many people spend up to ten thousand dollars a year on self-injectable growth-hormone therapy. You must decide if this for you, but with our exercise program you may not need it, especially if you are under age fifty. There is also a downside to artificially increasing your HGH level: increased insulin resistance, possible carpal tunnel syndrome, joint aches, and even edema (the accumulation of fluid in connective tissues) among women. Some doctors think that there is an increased cancer risk as well.

After just eight to ten seconds of 90 percent or more maximal high-intensity exercise, or twenty to thirty seconds of 70 to 90 percent maximal high-intensity exercise, your body will experience oxygen debt and an HGH release trigger. During recovery from this state, the body pays back the oxygen debt by increasing the heart rate and supplying oxygen to the blood with hard, rapid breathing. More than any other aspect of exercise, oxygen debt triggers HGH release.

Adults don't usually engage in the kind of intensity that shocks their bodies into this kind of growth stimulus. As a result they develop a slow-twitch crisis. Over the years they lose most of their fast-twitch and explosive fibers, which means that they can't get moving quickly, even though they may be able to run for hours at a time at a moderate pace. The good news is that these fibers don't disappear forever; they just become dormant. They are waiting to be reinvigorated.

Genetically, we are actually wired to do both fast and slow types of exertion and to have a significant explosive reserve with which to run, fight, or chase prey. Our modern world has removed us from that lifestyle, but our genetics have not changed in the past fifty thousand years, so our bodies maintain that capability.

Most adults have a low percentage of fast-twitch fibers, and it takes a while to reactivate them. With about six weeks of intense training, the fibers will redevelop; that's not a big investment of time to produce something that could result in a longer, healthier life span.

Why Aerobic Exercise Is Insufficient

The low-intensity exercise we think of as aerobics, or cardio training—for example, running on a treadmill for an hour while keeping your heart rate at 70 percent capacity—does not result in the same growth-hormone production as short bursts of intense physical work do. The reason is that your body is designed to avoid wasting energy, so it doesn't need to spend calories building muscle when the ones it has are doing perfectly well keeping you going at a moderate level of work.

Traditional endurance training involves primarily slow-twitch fibers that run on a combination of fat and oxygen. They do burn fat to make fuel, but the calories are burned at a much lower rate than with high-intensity exercise. For instance, if you burn five calories a minute, and all five of them are fat, that is great. But what if you burn twelve calories a minute, and eight of them are fat? You'd actually be burning more fat in less time, which is handy when your cell phone is trilling with new e-mails and you still have to hit the store to get something for dinner.

One very noticeable problem with aerobic exercise is that our fitness levels can plateau pretty rapidly, so the burning of fat slows down; we may be very efficient aerobic machines but still have more body fat than we'd like. This is one reason that people become frustrated with exercise and give up on it. No matter how long and how often they work out, they just don't seem to lose much weight.

We hope that you are now having an "Aha!" moment. Think about your current or most recent exercise program and why you probably had so much trouble getting rid of fat and building more endurance. You were most likely doing the wrong kind of exercise. The Immortality Edge fitness program will correct this rather quickly, and you'll smash through those plateaus of fitness and fat loss.

It's not just that our workout program will stimulate growth-hormone levels for a full two hours after you exercise. Studies show that short intense workouts are also great for turning on your metabolism and keeping it on for twenty-four hours or more after you have finished exercising. This is called *excess postexercise consumption*. Your metabolism is busy responding to the stress you caused with your intense workout for quite some time after the sweaty part is over.

One amazing study found that compared to runners of ten-kilometer races, people who practiced high-intensity training on a regular basis burned less than half the calories but up to nine times the body fat! The researchers were initially stumped by their findings. Why would people doing intense exercise burn fewer calories but more body fat?

As we now know, the answer is fairly obvious. Our metabolisms continue to operate at a faster rate long after the actual exercise period. The combined effect of naturally increased HGH secretion and the increased need to repair and recover from high-intensity workouts leads to incredible fat burning.

Thus, it's what happens after you are done working out that really matters. You become stronger, faster, leaner, and fitter as a result of the recovery or down time, not the actual exercise itself.

The process of recovery and repair also needs some nutritional help. Lots of protein—more than what is contained in the carbohydrate-rich diet that most of us consume—and enough vitamins and minerals help our cells to be efficient at repair. The right diet is essential, but many of the nutrients you need still have to come from supplements, as we noted in chapter 2.

Warming Up Is Not So Hard to Do

Our observation is that too many people don't warm up before they exercise. We see this all the time at the swimming pool: a middle-aged person jumps or dives into the water and immediately starts vigorous lap swimming. We see it at the gym: someone walks in and sits at the lateral pull-down machine and starts jerking a much too heavy weight up and down, thereby risking a serious shoulder injury. We see it at the tennis court: an elderly couple strolls out onto the court, and without doing even a single stretch, they start banging the ball back and forth from the baseline.

Why is this? Are most people in too big a hurry to warm up, are they too lazy, or are they just plain ignorant about the importance of warming up?

Warming up prevents injuries, and it makes for a better workout. It lubricates your joints, warms the connective tissues, activates your nervous system, and charges up your circulatory system. You should always do some simple stretches before you do any type of exercise, and you should always start out slowly and increase your speed over time.

Riding an exercise bike or running on a treadmill will get your heart pumping and cause you to sweat, but it won't properly warm you up for resistance training or weight lifting. The reason is that the related joints and connective tissues that you use for most resistance exercise (your elbows or shoulders, for example) are not activated during aerobic exercise. So if you immediately try to do some bicep hammer curls with a heavy weight, you are risking a muscle strain that could keep you out of the gym for a few weeks or more.

When doing resistance training, start with a low weight or resistance that allows you to do thirty or more repetitions, so that the specific muscles and joints being exercised can warm up. Do this first and then increase the weight or resistance so that you can do about fifteen repetitions. Increase it again

(continued)

(continued)

so that you can do ten or fewer. Gym instructors or personal trainers who tell you otherwise are unknowledgeable or under thirty or both; stay away from them.

When you go swimming, do a set of stretches (in or out of the water) that includes warming up your shoulders and stretching the muscles in your arms and legs as well as in your lower back. Begin your swim with a couple of slow laps and then increase the pace.

For tennis, you should do some stretching and then warm up by hitting the ball inside the service box for a few minutes. This is not only a safe way of getting your heart, lungs, muscles, and joints going, it is a good exercise in racket control.

Whatever the sport or activity, stretch first and start slowly. When you finish, don't just stop abruptly; let your body cool down gradually. Swim a couple of slow laps, hit a few lobs, or do some more stretches. Think of your body as a machine that will function better when it's properly cared for.

Telomeres and Your Workout

The telomere is like a biological clock that lives at the ends of our cells. It is vulnerable to the same stresses as all other genetic material. The primary toxin to the telomere is oxidation, which is often described as "body rust." This process is accelerated by the actions of free radicals, which are toxic forms of oxygen and nitrogen that in some circumstances are helpful on the cellular level by defending the immune system from invaders.

Some exercises are effective at preserving telomeres, but others are counterproductive. Certain sports and fitness practices create bodily stress by wearing out the tendons and the joints and by activating free radicals and the stress hormone cortisol. The repair process, in turn, creates another problem: cell replication rapidly increases, and each time a cell replicates, its telomere loses some of its DNA base pairs. In other words, it gets shorter.

Athletes who participate in extreme sports (including marathons, triathlons, and long-distance cycling) and in violent sports (such as football or boxing) are fooling themselves if they think that their activities will extend their life spans. The strained knees, stress fractures, bad backs, and other routine injuries that nearly all of them suffer, and the concussions and broken bones endured by participants in violent sports, are only the tip of the iceberg when it comes to self-inflicted damage.

Numerous studies have found that cardiac injury can be seen after prolonged, strenuous exercise. A recent Harvard study of Boston Marathon runners found that nearly all of them suffer some heart damage—indeed, some marathon runners actually drop dead from cardiac arrest during or shortly after a race. It is also common knowledge that football players and boxers often develop long-term brain damage (witness Muhammad Ali) and severe arthritis.

The programs in the Immortality Edge are skewed toward high-intensity noncardio kinds of training. We want you to make exercise a priority in your life, but in order to make this easier for you, our program requires only half (or less) of the time commitment of most traditional programs while providing at least twice the benefit.

What about Yoga?

You don't have to start yoga classes to follow the Immortality Edge fitness program, but yoga is fantastic and highly recommended. If you're already doing yoga, don't stop—not that you'd want to!

Yoga improves flexibility, muscular strength, and balance, and even if meditation is not part of the style of yoga you practice, it definitely provides some relief from everyday stress. Nevertheless, it's not a good idea to depend on yoga as your sole form of exercise, because it does little to improve aerobic fitness, it isn't at all anaerobic, and it doesn't burn many calories. (Unless you are an advanced practitioner of Ashtanga or Power Yoga.) A fifty-minute session of hatha yoga burns approximately 140 calories, about the number you would find in a couple of carrots.

One of the really important benefits of yoga is that it strengthens the lower back muscles. Research at the University of Washington found that people with chronic back pain got more relief from yoga than from doing traditional exercises designed by a physical therapist. If you have back pain, however, don't just sign up for the nearest yoga class. It could be too strenuous and end up causing you more pain. Look instead for a therapeutic yoga class that has been designed to deal with back problems.

We are huge proponents of yoga because it not only stretches the body in the ways that have proven beneficial for thousands of years, but it also calms the mind and provides a mind-body connection that is truly magical. "You are using your whole body on different planes and rotations," yoga pioneer Baron Baptiste said in an article published in *Ms. Fitness* magazine. "It's strength and flexibility building for everyday life."

Baptiste is the creator of Baptiste Power Vinyasa Yoga (www.baronbaptiste.com) and has been practicing and teaching for decades. "Mentally, we go through life soaking up stresses like a sponge," he said in the same interview. "Stress blocks energy. Doing a rigorous yoga wrings out your sponge leaving you feeling clear and puts you into that calm eye of the storm ridding you of the poisons and pressures of everyday life. Yoga is like Mylanta for the mind."

If practiced incorrectly, however, yoga can do more damage to the body than good. Misaligned poses can lead to injuries ranging from aching joints to pulled muscles. "Yoga injuries are often a result of not knowing or realizing your body's limitations," says yoga instructor and educational kinesiologist Candace Morano of New York City (www.explorevidyayoga.com). "This goes for beginners and advanced students, as some beginners under-estimate how strenuous yoga can be, and some who are more advanced overestimate their strength and flexibility."

A glance at the daily schedule of an Equinox Fitness club in New York City proves the availability and variety of yoga classes offered at leading facilities. The schedule has everything from Hatha Yoga and Warrior Flow Yoga to Vinyasa Yoga and Sacred Strength Flow Yoga. There is a style and intensity of yoga for all levels of interest and fitness.

If you are one of those people who say, "I'm stiff as a board and can't stretch" or "I've lost all of the flexibility I had as a kid," take heart. The benefits of stretching do not belong only to the limber, Gumby bodies of the world. In fact, you will have to work *less* to get more benefit, since a very limber person will have to go very deep and work very hard to "feel" what you are feeling on day one. Also, you will begin to see improvement within just a few sessions.

Max Strom's bio tells us that he "founded and directed the renowned Sacred Movement Center for Yoga and Healing in Los Angeles." There he taught more than four hundred students a week for over four years, building the program into one of the most respected centers in the world. In 2005, he sold the studio to Exhale Spa, which continues to thrive. He has taught tens of thousands of students; trained several hundred teachers; and recorded two videos, *Learn to Breathe, to Heal Yourself and Your Relationships* and *Max Strom Yoga—Strength, Grace, Healing*. His book *A Life Worth Breathing: A Yoga Master's Handbook of Strength, Grace and Healing*, about the far-reaching benefits of yoga, is beautifully written and inspiring.

Make it a priority to go to the gym and take that first stretching or beginning yoga class. Buy an instructional DVD on stretching or yoga. (We recommend any product offered by Baron Baptiste or Bryan Kest of www.poweryoga.com. Both are extraordinary teachers and offer instructional DVDs that can be used by any-one, beginner to advanced, as a regular part of a powerful fitness program.)

The Stretch toward Immortality

Why is it that you can calculate if a person is young or old simply by watching him or her walk down the street from afar? After all, you cannot see from a distance the facial features (wrinkles, sagging skin, age spots, and the like) that are age cues. You cannot speak to the person to determine his or her maturity and wisdom—or lack thereof. Yet a teenager is easily distinguished from an octogenarian from a few blocks away.

Part of the reason lies in the mobility and grace with which a person moves. Someone who is bent over or walking rigidly and slowly looks very different from a person who is moving with ease and grace. Part of this difference lies not in an aging genome but in a body that has not been allowed to flourish and thrive through daily stretching movements of some kind.

Stretching is a key part of longevity and vitality, because it can help you to lose weight through the firing of muscle fibers that allow you to go deeper into your exercises during workouts, pumping up the heart rate and burning more calories. When you increase your range of motion, your balance improves, and you are less likely to fall. Increased blood flow to the muscles through stretching improves circulation. Your posture will improve through the better body alignment that stretching provides, and you will not have the octogenarian look when you are viewed from a distance.

Increased mobility and range of motion makes daily life better. Everything becomes easier, from walking the dog to taking out the trash to running up a flight of stairs to catch an airplane.

Stretching involves anything that you do on a regular basis that takes the body through a range of motions and, in doing so, restores equilibrium and reduces stress. Yoga and Pilates are two forms of stretching that are hugely popular today. Yoga, especially, provides much more than just a means to lengthen and release the body, but its benefits in that area are truly regenerative.

There are many other ways, old and new, to keep the body fluid and mobile. Active Isolated Stretching (AIS), for example, is a relatively new protocol that is proving beneficial and is used in health care, sports, and massage and by physical therapists, chiropractors, osteopaths, athletic trainers, and athletes. It varies from more conventional methods because the stretches are held for no more than two seconds rather than the sixty seconds of many other styles. Its proponents cite its ability to increase full range of motion from head to toe and its neuromuscular reeducation, which trains the body to be flexible.

Working your own Immortality Edge fitness program will not be complete without some form of regular stretching. Find a technique that allows you to explore and expand on a daily basis, even for just a few minutes a day. Soon you'll find that your day goes better with a bit of bend in it.

Resistance Training

As with yoga, if you are lifting weights or doing other forms of strength or resistance training, we want you to continue doing this. If you are not, you should seriously consider adding strength training to your workout schedule.

You're never too old to pump iron. Even if you are in your nineties, you can become stronger—a good resistance training program will increase your strength by 25 to 100 percent or more within one year. In contrast, a good aerobic exercise program will increase your aerobic fitness by only 15 to 25 percent.

The "resistance" in resistance training comes from pitting the muscles against a force, usually a dumbbell or a barbell. Body weight itself can provide the resistance: pull-ups, sit-ups, and push-ups are a form of resistance training. Isometric exercises, in which you push your hands against a doorway or against the opposing limb of an exercise partner, are another example. Bands, free weights, and resistance machines are by far the best methods.

How does resistance training work? Basically, the cells in your muscles adapt to the extra workload by enlarging (thus the term *pumped up*) and by subsequently recruiting nerve cells to contract themselves. After a muscle has been subjected to intense stress through maximal-force contractions over a moderate repetition range, hormones begin the growth process and muscle remodeling. Like the interval training we advocate, resistance training can increase growth-hormone levels.

When using free weights or resistance machines, use a weight that allows eight to twelve repetitions before maximum voluntary contraction sets in. This means that your muscle has contracted to its peak. If fact, you should feel a burning sensation in your arm as you do the final repetition—this is good. If you do three sets of eight to twelve repetitions using the maximum amount of weight and you rest for only sixty seconds or less between sets, your muscles will release the maximum amount of hormones. They will grow in size and capacity (strength). This is so amazingly simple that we wonder why so many people at the gym don't do it our way.

A Final Thought on Aerobic Exercise

Before we move on to the specifics of the Immortality Edge fitness program, we want to be clear that although we advocate high-intensity interval training, plain aerobic exercise is still much better than not exercising at all or just walking around the neighborhood once in awhile.

We hope that you'll plunge into our program in chapter 7, but even if you stick to jogging, swimming, cycling, or vigorous walking, you'll still delay biological aging, just not as much.

Aerobic power typically declines with age. The average sixty-year-old has only half the capacity to take in and use oxygen as a twenty-year-old. If you do regular aerobic exercise, you can reduce this decline by 80 percent. That's not bad, but according to the latest findings published in the *British Journal of Sports Medicine*, high-intensity aerobic exercise can actually boost your aerobic power by 25 percent in one year. And if you stay aerobically fit throughout your middle years and into your elderly years, you can delay biological aging by up to twelve years.

4

The Immortality Edge
Stress-Reduction Plan

Meditation can be the ticket to reducing your stress while lengthening your telomeres. Here's an irrefutably true scientific statement: chronic stress over time accelerates cellular aging. Nobel Prize winner Elizabeth Blackburn, PhD, first uncovered this fact in 2004 with the publication of her monumental research on sixty-two premenopausal biological mothers, ages twenty to fifty. In the control group, each mother had a healthy child, and in the experimental group, each mother had a chronically ill child. For a number of years, the women were tested and retested for their stress levels and for the rate of aging of their cells measured by white blood cell tests. These tests measured the length of their telomeres as well as two other biomarkers of cellular aging: telomerase activity and oxidative stress. The results were stunning.

In both groups of mothers, the researchers found that the higher the perceived stress, the faster the rate of cellular aging and telomere shortening, and the number of years of caregiving related to how much shorter the telomeres became. Indeed, the telomere shortening in the high-stress mothers was equivalent to nine to seventeen years of extra aging.

This established a definite correlation between stress and cellular aging, but does it prove causality? Along with measuring the aging biomarkers, Blackburn also measured the levels of three chronic stress hormones: cortisol, epinephrine, and norepinephrine. Sure enough, the levels of these hormones went up in lockstep with the rate of telomere shortening, a decline of telomerase activity, and an increase in oxidation. "Chronic stress is what is wearing down the telomeres," Blackburn said recently in a public lecture at the University of California–San Francisco titled "Stress, Telomeres and Telomerase in Humans."

These days, Professor Blackburn is interested is finding out if meditation can slow the rate of cellular aging as well as the rate of cognitive decline. In a preliminary finding, she has reported, "Given the pattern of associations revealed so far, we propose [that] some forms of meditation may have salutary effects on telomere length by reducing cognitive stress and stress arousal and increasing positive states of mind and hormonal factors that may promote telomere maintenance. Aspects of this model are currently being tested in ongoing trials of mindfulness meditation."

We have noticed over the years the tendency of many scientists, most especially Blackburn, to be exceedingly cautious in the conclusions they make about their own research. We strongly suspect that the phrase "some forms of meditation may have salutary effects on telomere length" will turn out to be a perfect example. Our expectation is that when the results are in, the word *salutary* will accurately be replaced with the word *profound*.

The Power of Meditation

"Mindfulness Meditation" is one of many types of meditation used by practitioners looking for that all-important mind-body connection. It emphasizes an immediate awareness of your experience in all areas of activity by, essentially, concentrating your mind on the present. To practice this, you sit bolt upright with intense alertness, attending to the flow or to ordinary and usually banal and sometimes uncomfortable phenomena such as itches, sounds, thought patterns, and tensions.

Mindfulness meditation is very different from the classic mantra meditation, including Transcendental Meditation (TM), that is probably more familiar to Westerners, but it is growing in

A Little Zen Will Do You

As we were writing this book, a significant study appeared in *Consciousness and Cognition*, an international science journal. The psychologists found, to their amazement, that students who meditated for just four days showed significant improvement in their cognitive skills. The sixty-three students who took part in this experiment were randomly assigned to one of two groups. The first group received mindfulness meditation training while the other group listened for equivalent amounts of time to J. R. R. Tolkien's book *The Hobbit* being read aloud.

The cognitive skills of both groups were measured before and after by a broad battery of behavioral tests that assessed mood, memory, visual attention, attention processing, and vigilance. At the beginning, the two groups performed equally. On the second test, the first group improved slightly, whereas the meditation group scored consistently higher on every measure. On the tests that involved the ability to concentrate while holding other information in mind, the meditation group scored as much as ten times higher.

One of the researchers, Professor Fadel Zeidan, said, "Findings like these suggest [that] meditation's benefits may not require extensive training to be realized and that meditation's first benefits may be associated with increasing the ability to sustain attention."

popularity in both Europe and the United States. In TM, you sit comfortably, hands resting on your legs, eyes closed, and silently repeat a mantra for up to twenty minutes, twice a day. It is relatively easy and usually brings immediate calming effects.

There are other popular styles of meditation, including the relaxation response, but it probably doesn't matter which style is used. The result of any successful meditation is to achieve deeper and deeper levels of calmness, relaxation, and concentration, sometimes referred to as an altered state of consciousness or nirvana.

Practicing meditation does not mean you have to become a spiritual person, a Zen Buddhist, or a Tibetan monk. None of those things is bad, but meditation is really about something else: fulfilling the capacity we have as humans to become more present in our lives, calmer, more purposeful, and more aware. Some would say that meditation is about awakening us to the power within, the ability we have to steer ourselves more peacefully through whatever troubled water lies ahead. If it brings along a dose of unintended spiritual enlightenment, consider that a bonus.

For our purposes, meditation is the antidote to stress. Its life-prolonging and transforming power comes from its ability to undo the significant damage, including telomere damage, that we suffer from our crazy, mixed-up, overstimulated, unpredictable, pressure-cooker, so-called modern lifestyle. Meditation brings about decreased muscle tension, lowered heart rate and blood pressure, a deeper breathing pattern, an inner calm, and a peaceful, pleasant mood.

Until recently, the benefits of meditation were thought to be a self-delusion or highly exaggerated, because there was no real way to prove that they actually provoked any kind of physical response. In the last decade, however, there has been a resurgence of scientific research on meditation because of the wide availability of increasingly sophisticated brain-scanning technology.

In one such study, University of California–Los Angeles (UCLA) psychologists hooked up two groups of students to functional magnetic resonance imaging (fMRI) machines, which scan the brain to reveal which parts are active and inactive at any given moment. The people in the first group regularly practiced mindfulness meditation, and those in the second group did not. After asking the participants to complete questionnaires to describe their present emotions, thoughts, and sensations without reacting strongly to them, the researchers compared the brain scans and found a stark difference. The meditating group experienced far greater activation in the right prefrontal cortex and a greater calming effect in the amygdala after labeling their emotions. Here was the physical evidence the psychologists were looking for: meditation really does give practitioners the ability to examine emotional matters in a detached manner.

At the University of Wisconsin, scientists used brain scanners to compare newly trained meditators to people with up to fifty-four thousand hours of meditation experience. All of the subjects underwent an fMRI scan while meditating. All those in the experienced group had much greater activity in the brain circuits that relate to paying attention and making decisions. Isolating only those with at least forty thousand hours of experience produced an even more profound result. After showing a brief increase in brain activity when the subjects started meditating, the brain wave scans came down to the baseline. It was as though these meditators were able to concentrate in a totally effortless way. And guess what: effortless concentration is a characteristic of advanced meditation that is often described in classic meditation books, some of which preceded fMRI scanning by centuries.

The UCLA and University of Wisconsin studies are just two examples of hundreds of studies that validate the many claimed benefits of meditation. Many of these benefits have a direct bearing on longevity. In researching this book, we challenged ourselves to see if we couldn't find at least fifty proven ways in which meditation prolongs life, in addition to, or in conjunction with, helping to maintain telomeres. It wasn't too hard.

Fifty Ways in Which the Practice of Meditation Prolongs Life

1. Exercises the critical prefrontal cortex of the brain
2. Increases blood flow by dilating the blood vessels
3. Lowers blood pressure
4. Increases the serotonin level
5. Lowers the level of blood lactate, thus reducing anxiety
6. Improves the efficiency of oxygen consumption
7. Decreases the respiratory rate while increasing lung capacity
8. Leads to deeper levels of relaxation and, consequently, deeper sleep
9. Decreases muscle tension
10. Reduces premenstrual syndrome symptoms
11. Improves the brain's executive function
12. Increases working memory
13. Reduces impulsive behavior
14. Produces a state of restful alertness
15. Reduces the activation of the sympathetic nervous system, thus counteracting stress
16. Reduces the thickening of coronary arteries
17. Slows or stops the progression of atherosclerosis
18. Boosts the immune system
19. Lowers the LDL ("bad") cholesterol level
20. Increases perceptual ability
21. Creates detachment from emotional events
22. Increases the ability to solve complex problems
23. Increases brain wave coherence
24. Reduces the time it takes to fall asleep
25. Harmonizes the endocrine system
26. Provides significant relief to asthma sufferers
27. Stimulates the pituitary gland to produce higher levels of DHEA
28. Controls pain
29. Reduces free radicals
30. Increases exercise tolerance

31. Reduces societal stress, crime, and violence when practiced in groups
32. Increases happiness
33. Speeds up reaction time
34. Increases social tolerance
35. Lowers the risk of diabetes
36. Reduces or eliminates negative thoughts
37. Increases the melatonin level
38. Lowers cortisol
39. Boosts endorphins
40. Shifts brain waves in the stress-prone right frontal cortex to the calmer left frontal cortex
41. Minimizes brain activity in the amygdala, where the brain processes fear
42. Decreases anxiety and depression
43. Increases clarity while reducing confusion
44. Resolves digestive problems
45. Brings about a high level of self-acceptance
46. Lowers stroke risk
47. Increases self-reflectiveness
48. Heightens all senses
49. Loosens the hold of addictions
50. Balances the physical, mental, and emotional states

TM Lowers the Rates of Heart Attack, Stroke, and Death by 50 Percent and Enhances Brain Function

A first-ever study on meditation to be presented at a meeting of the American Heart Association found that patients with narrowing of the arteries in their hearts—average age, fifty-nine years—who practiced TM had nearly 50 percent lower rates of heart attack, stroke, and death, compared to a nonmeditating

(continued)

(continued)

group. Other studies recently published in the neuroscience journal *Cognitive Processing* show that brain development can be enhanced—not only during adolescence but at any age—through the Transcendental Meditation technique, and that different meditation techniques have different effects on the brain.

Aleta St. James Spreads the Power of Meditation

Imagine a life-changing concert that combines elements of the rock opera *Tommy*, Peter Gabriel, and the best of the world music experience. That is where you will find Aleta St. James leading audiences as she spreads her healing work beyond the realm of life coaching in private sessions. For thirty years she has been a renowned energy healer, success coach, and top-selling author of *Life Shift: Let Go and Live Your Dream*. Aleta, sixty-three, proves that life really begins to peak after fifty. Her extraordinary healing gifts are why celebrities like Carolyn Murphy, Lori Petty, and Taylor Dayne, and leading fashion designers like Todd Oldham flock to her.

In 2004, at age fifty-seven, Aleta broke through the glass ceiling of motherhood. Her story made headlines around the world; she became a sought-after guest on television, attracting TV anchors like Diane Sawyer and Katie Couric, who have featured her on their newscasts. Aleta's gorgeous twins, Gian and Francesca, are now six years old. Not that any of this was exactly what Aleta saw for herself when she was younger, but she says it's all about "letting go of what you thought the dream was and how you are going to get it, and enjoying what the dream is."

One of the key tools in her arsenal as she does battle with people's personal challenges is the teaching of meditation practice. She, like the authors of this book, believes that mediation and mindfulness can add years to our biological clocks and unleash creativity to enrich those years. She spoke to us for the purposes of this book and shared her insights:

Meditation activates and regenerates the life force energy of your body, mind, and spirit. I've seen incredible changes, transformations, and healing in thousands of my clients throughout the world.

All of your past experiences, your belief systems, what you have accepted as truth—all of these combined help you see the world through either a positive or negative filter. If your filters are mostly negative, you're likely experiencing stress, anxiety, and depression that's taking a toll on your relationships, financial situation, health, and quality of life.

Active meditation goes to the core or root of what's creating this negativity, eliminates the cause, and allows you to have the life you want and deserve.

For example, I had a client who on the surface looked like she should be on top of the world. She was young, beautiful, and tremendously talented. But as she pursued a show business career, nothing seemed to work out. She would go into auditions and freeze up. Parts would go to other less talented actresses or performers. She was beside herself. Though she said her positive affirmations every day, on a deep level, she didn't believe it.

In desperation, she tried my meditation techniques. Through the techniques of conscious breathing, the healing power of light, she was able to get in touch what was really going on inside. During one meditation, she discovered that she was holding on to criticism she received from her mother every time she tried to show her creativity. "Who do you think you are, no one wants to hear you sing? Who would want to listen to you?"

(continued)

(continued)

It turns out her mother had aspirations of her own to perform but got married early and had to give them up, never following her dream. That strong messaging made my client shut down in auditions, because she subconsciously had accepted her mother's message that no one *did* want to hear her sing or perform.

But through the practice of meditation she was able to release those feelings, shift her focus, and land some parts. Eventually, she even made it to Broadway. She's now a flourishing actress and musical stage performer who's in full charge of her gifts.

Meditation is also amazing for shifting into vibrant health. Stress limits the cells of our body's ability to regenerate and be healthy, because instead of your natural healing energy being in full flow, that energy is taken up in a "fight or flight" mode, taxing valuable resources that should be focusing on your natural state of peace, health, well-being and vitality.

For instance, you've seen people who are happy, content, and accepting and are filled with energy and a natural zest for living. This is our natural state when we are self-accepting and in full flow of higher source energy.

Meditation can help get to the root cause of your negative thoughts and emotions that create negative stress, release them, and then create your dreams, hopes, and desires without old resistance.

You are constantly in a state of clearing and shifting negative mental and emotional energy and putting yourself in a state of creativity and possibility, so that you experience a sense of authentic empowerment. In this positive state, your cells will actually move, rearrange, and communicate this into a place of calmness, vibrancy, inner peace, and well-being. Creative possibility suddenly becomes a reality.

The key to youth and vitality is not just dealing with your physical body, there's another very important—essential, in fact—component that works in concert to help keep you young and vibrant. Your emotional state needs tending as well.

Meditation and Sleep: The Immortality Edge Relax and Rejuvenate Your Telomeres Technique

Hundreds of thousands of people worldwide are dying each year because of undiagnosed and untreated sleep disorders.

Meditation is one answer to this problem. Researchers have found that people who meditate regularly sleep longer and more deeply than those who don't meditate, and the reason isn't simply that they are more relaxed. Nor does it matter whether you meditate just before going to bed. Regular meditation increases the level of two important hormones, serotonin and melatonin, while decreasing the level of a third, cortisol. Serotonin, the happiness hormone, reduces everyday anxiety; melatonin helps to control your natural sleep-wake cycle; and cortisol, as we have mentioned several times, is the main stress hormone.

The added bonus of meditation is that you are more restful during the day and, consequently, get more rest and deeper sleep at night. All this adds up to less stress on a cellular level, longer telomeres, and a longer life.

Now, time to begin to meditate, Immortality Edge style. As we've explained, there are myriad ways to de-stress, meditate, relax, and unwind. The key to refreshing your mind and rejuvenating your telomeres, however, is to practice something, almost anything, on a regular, if not *daily*, basis. By utilizing a relaxation practice regularly you can help to counteract all of the deleterious effects of stress, which cannot be totally avoided. They're a part of life in this day and age; there's no getting around it.

The relax and rejuvenate (R&R) technique is a simple way to access this healing practice for those who do not currently meditate or pray regularly. It can be done anytime or anywhere but we recommend that it be done *every day*.

For starters, you may be able to carve out the bandwidth or time for only a few minutes a day. That is perfect. By sticking with it and gradually lengthening the time you spend doing this critical exercise, you will reap benefits that will exponentially improve your healthspan and quality of life. Eventually, you may find that your day just doesn't go right if you don't take this time out for yourself. Following are the steps to practice R&R.

Step One: Alternate Nostril Breathing

Begin by finding a quiet place for yourself at home, at the office, or wherever. If you do this at home and you live with others, tell them that you are taking some important quiet time for yourself and ask not to be disturbed, if at all possible. Distractions will crop up, but you will get better over time at tuning them out or dealing with them—if you must—and then going back to your quiet time.

Pick a spot that is peaceful and makes you feel relaxed rather than anxious. You may light a candle or incense if that helps you get in that relaxed mood that you are seeking.

First, and most important, turn off phones, lower the volume on computers that sound off with alarms of any kind, and kill the TV set for this important time.

You don't have to turn out the lights or draw the curtains unless any light flooding in is very distracting.

Close any doors or windows that allow in noises that will be overly distracting to you. (Jackhammers on the street cannot be stopped, but if you can, close the window—it might help you to focus inward.)

Find a comfortable seated position and just let your hands fall naturally onto the tops of your legs. Relax.

Close your eyes and begin to breathe a bit more deeply, closing your mouth and inhaling and exhaling through your nose.

Place your right hand near your nose, and as you inhale, close the left nostril off with your ring finger and breathe in, counting slowly to seven.

At the top of the inhale place your right thumb against your right nostril, closing off the breath. Hold for a count of seven.

Release the ring finger and exhale through the left nostril, this time to a slow fourteen count.

At the bottom of the exhale immediately breathe in again through the left nostril, still blocking the right nostril with the right thumb.

At the top of the inhale again block both nostrils and count to seven.

Release the right thumb and exhale through the right nostril to the count of fourteen, keeping the block on the left nostril with the ring finger.

Repeat by inhaling through the right nostril to the same slow seven count and holding at the top as you did in the first round.

Perform seven complete rounds of this and end on a right nostril exhale.

Step Two: Long Spine Breathing

After you have completed ten rounds of alternate nostril breathing relax for a few normal breaths and place your hands once again on your legs or lap.

Next, draw a deep breath in and visualize it beginning at the base of your spine. As you inhale, visualize a ball of white light moving slowly up your spine with the breath.

As the breath enters your brain, imagine that the ball of white light expands, filling the brain completely.

Exhale, and as you do, shrink down the visualized ball of white light so that it can begin the trip down toward the base of your spine.

When the breath and the visualized ball of white light reach the base of your spine start the inhale again and repeat. Perform this visualization seven times.

Step Three: Go Deep Inside

Once you have performed the alternate nostril breathing and the long spine inhale you are ready to spend as much time as you have left to simply do *nothing*. Continue to breathe in and out through the nose. Find a spot within, whether it is the much talked about Third Eye (between the eyes, on the forehead) or your heart center. This will be your Relaxation Center.

Keep your focus on your breath and the Relaxation Center. Thoughts will come and go. There is no stopping the chatter that goes on in the busy human brain. Simply notice the thoughts and release them with the breath.

Ideally, you will spend a total of about eighteen to twenty minutes each day on your Immortality Edge R&R sessions. If at first all you can manage to do is the alternate nostril breathing or the spine breath or both, great. Do what you can and build up to a total time of eighteen to twenty minutes. Even two minutes on your first try is a start. As the Nike advertisements say, Just Do It.

Many people complain that they simply can't afford time for meditation or downtime. To the contrary, when it comes to your health span and your telomeres, you can't afford *not* to take the time to restore them.

Others worry that they are not doing it right. There is no way to do this practice wrong. If you find yourself focusing on the problems of the day or a challenge you are facing, that is fine and perfectly normal. When you find yourself straying from your Relaxation Center bring yourself back with the breath.

There will be days when you go blissfully blank and days when you cannot stop the chatter. Both are fine. You are doing tremendous good for yourself and getting benefit in both cases and with everything in between.

Remember, the secret is in consistency.

If you are interrupted during your R&R session—and, as we have seen over the years, interruptions will happen— ask the person demanding your attention if you can have another ten minutes to finish your R&R and then deal with the issue. Or if you *must* interrupt your R&R to solve a real emergency, do so as quickly as possible and then get back to your R&R as soon as you appropriately can and begin again.

Stealing away for only five to ten minutes on your busiest day is a necessity for another important reason. Finding that quick calm in the midst of insanity may make the difference between health and disease over the long haul.

5

Add Years to Your Life

Let's review a few basic concepts about telomeres and how they are affected by our lifestyle choices.

A Quick Review of Telomere Concepts

- Telomeres are the biological clocks that are ticking from the day we are conceived until the day we die.
- When cells divide and replicate, we lose telomere length. Cellular reproduction is required on a regular basis to repair damaged tissue and to cope with stresses, both good and bad.
- When telomeres are reduced to approximately five thousand base pairs, our cells become senescent and die. For this reason, the maximum life span until now has been 120 years. Only one person in human history has been documented to have lived longer than this (122 years).

- Smoking, drinking, sleep deprivation, chronic stress, illnesses, hormonal imbalance, sedentary behavior, obesity, exposure to environmental toxins, and injury all increase the cellular replicative process, which in turn speeds up telomere loss.

- Controlling free radicals, oxidation, glycation, and methylation slows down telomere shortening. Eating well, getting adequate sleep, exercising regularly (the type recommended in this book), meditating, and taking the right supplements accomplishes these things. Therefore, telomere preservation is available to everyone.

- Shorter than normal telomeres are associated with the diseases of aging, including heart disease, Alzheimer's disease, osteoporosis, and arthritis.

- There are mechanisms in our bodies to stop sick, mutated, and dying cells from reproducing. If these mechanisms are somehow bypassed, the telomerase gene can be over-expressed, causing a huge increase in the telomerase enzyme, which creates an immortal cell line that is not subject to normal growth controls. This then becomes cancer.

- Paradoxically, lengthening the telomeres of healthy cells helps to prevent cancer and other diseases by boosting the immune system and making the genome (the DNA) more stable.

- Lengthening the telomeres also extends the life span of the cells and ultimately of the organism.

- There are telomerase activators available, including TA-65, which will lengthen telomeres. Other activators and telomere inducers are in development. Full-fledged telomere therapy should be available within the next decade.

Testing for Telomeres

Now that we have reviewed the basics, just how do you have your telomeres measured?

Any physician may order telomere testing. The standard test is called a polymerase chain reaction (PCR) test. It involves a simple blood test in which about two tablespoons of blood are drawn. Most testing is done by SpectraCell, a laboratory in Houston, Texas. The cost, as of this writing, is $350.

The SpectraCell PCR test can determine the median length of your telomeres in relation to your age. It is calculated by taking the average, or mean telomere length (MTL), of the telomeres in your white blood cells (T-lymphocytes) and then comparing this to the MTLs from a broad sample of the U.S. population in your age range. The higher the telomere score, the younger the cells. It's pretty simple.

There are some problems with MTL testing, however. If you measured your telomeres now and saved some extra blood samples for future testing, the same test on your stored blood six months from now should produce the same results. However, if you draw more blood in six months and test it again using the same procedure, the same lab, and even the same lab technicians, you will probably get a significantly different result.

This different result won't make much sense, because the normal changes that telomeres undergo are too small to see much, if any, change in this short time. The reason is that it is nearly impossible to get the perfect blood sample in which the telomeres of the white blood cells are truly average. Each sample is only an approximation.

The solution for people who want to keep track of the rate of their telomere shortening, or who want to see if their telomeres have grown longer because they are taking a telomere activator like TA-65, is to draw multiple tubes of blood (usually up to seven), test one, and freeze the rest at minus forty-seven degrees Fahrenheit for later testing. This lets your doctor or lab analyst directly compare the telomere lengths of any new test with those of the first test.

The MTL data comparing one test to another are more useful the longer you wait—one or even two years is best. The telomere of an average cell of a normally aging human loses approximately forty base pairs per year, and even an accelerated loss of a hundred base pairs is not easy to detect. One drawback to repeat-diagnostic telomere testing is that the cost goes up to about $900. Also, having seven tubes of blood drawn at one time can cause anxiety for some people.

Still, repeat-diagnostic testing remains the current gold standard for people who want to monitor the effects of taking telomerase activators.

The PCR test we've been discussing isn't the only type of telomere testing; there are two more. One is called the *flow-FISH test* and the other is called *short telomere testing*.

The flow-FISH (fluorescence in situ hybridization) test involves a complicated process of cloning the telomere gene, painting it with a fluorescent dye, and then mapping it to a chromosome. Not yet widely available and prohibitively expensive, the flow-FISH test provides scientists with an accurate way of measuring telomere length and the percentage of short telomeres in large human sample sets. It is currently being used to uncover associations between telomere length and human disease.

As of this writing, short telomere testing was available at only one lab, in Spain, where it is being used strictly as a research tool. This will certainly change. Because of the huge importance of telomere testing and the surging demand, scientists and entrepreneurs are partnering to find ways to make this test widely available and affordable.

Short telomere testing could turn out to be the more valuable of the two, because research by Nobel Prize winner Carol Greider at Johns Hopkins University indicates that it is actually the single shortest telomere in a cell that controls its fate. "Our evidence suggests that once a telomere becomes very short, the cell recognizes it as a DNA break," Greider notes. "Broken DNA commonly signals normal cells to arrest or die as a protection against chromosome rearrangement and cancer."

In tests on mice, scientists have determined that telomerase activators save cells by lengthening only the shortest telomeres

Reinforcing Your Body's Tumor Immune Surveillance System

Your immune system has three powerful ways by which to prevent the development of cancer. First, by eliminating or suppressing viral infections, it protects you from virus-induced cancers. Second, the timely elimination of pathogens and the prompt resolution of inflammation prevents the establishment of an inflammatory environment, which is conducive to the development of tumors. Third, the most remarkable method, your immune system specifically identifies and kills tumor cells based on their expression of tumor-specific antigens, or molecules induced by cellular stress.

This third process is known as *tumor immune surveillance*. Your immune system identifies cancerous and precancerous cells and eliminates them before they can cause harm. If this weren't the case, human beings probably would have been wiped out many generations ago, because all of our bodies develop some cancerous and precancerous cells.

We do know that people with a chronic viral infection known as CMV (cytomegalovirus) which infects up to 30 percent of the general population, respond to TA-65 with increasing white blood cell counts, indicating a strengthening of the immune system. As of this writing there is no other comercially available compound that does this. CMV is often considered a marker for "immunosenescence or aging of the immune system," which is in turn considered to be an increased risk for cancer and death.

It is far too early to say with certainty, but there is great hope for further cancer reduction in immune-boosting compounds like the telomerase activator TA-65. Telomerase inhibitors will no doubt be used to restore mortality to immortal cancer cells, but telomerase activators may prevent cancer in the first place by reinforcing the body's tumor immune surveillance system. It's a rather interesting paradox!

rather than acting on them indiscriminately. In terms of survival, this makes sense, since the longer telomeres are not causing any problems and do not need to be fixed—a marvelous example of how efficient an enzyme system can be at doing only what is necessary.

The Complete Telomere Age Test

We urge you to arrange with your doctor to get the basic $350 PCR test and to at least consider the more expensive repeat-diagnostic testing. Telomere length is the only truly accurate biomarker of aging available, and knowing where you stand could be a crucial step on the path to living a much longer, healthier life.

Meanwhile, we've devised a simple test you can take yourself that will give you an approximation of your telomere age and also provide you with plenty of clues about things you can do right now to start down the very long road of infinite longevity.

The questions on our test are based on known illnesses, conditions, and behaviors that correlate with telomere length. All three of us have had our telomere lengths tested, and we've taken this test; the results were within a few years for each of us!

What's Your Telomere Age?

You'll need a calculator or a long sheet of paper and a pen or a pencil. Start with ten thousand points and add or subtract points as directed after answering each question. If you prefer, you can add up your results at the end.

1. Starting with your chronological age, subtract 250 points for every decade over age twenty. For example, if you are fifty years old, that's three decades over age twenty. Subtract 750 (3 × 250) from 10,000 and move on to the next question.

2. Do you smoke, or have you ever smoked, cigarettes? If yes, subtract 250 points for every decade you smoked more than five cigarettes a day.
3. Do you currently drink more than two drinks of alcohol a day or more than twelve fluid ounces in a week? If so, subtract 250 points.
4. Do you binge drink? Subtract 250 points.
5. Do you use recreational drugs? Deduct 100 points for marijuana and 200 for cocaine, LSD, methamphetamine, or heroin. If you use more than one recreational drug, subtract 300 points.
6. On most nights, do you sleep less than five hours or more than nine hours? Think back, then subtract 50 points for every decade you've had this sleep pattern.
7. Do you have sleep apnea? If so, subtract another 100 points. (Sleep is the most underrated anti-aging tool. Proper hormone regulation and secretion is tied to proper sleep.)
8. Do you have high blood pressure? Deduct 200 points if it is not controlled.
9. Do you have diabetes? If your diabetes is under control, subtract 100 points. If not, subtract 250.
10. If you are more than ten pounds overweight, subtract 50 points.
11. If you are more than thirty pounds overweight, subtract an additional 200 points.
12. Have you gained more than ten pounds per decade since turning thirty? Sorry, but if so, subtract 50 points. (A sure sign of both hormonal aging and a sedentary lifestyle is steady weight gain over each decade of life after age thirty. It signifies decreased strength and, of course, increased fat, unless you happen to be a bodybuilder and your weight gain is mostly muscle.)
13. If you are male and your waist measurement is greater than thirty-six inches, subtract 50 points. If you are female and

your waist is more than thirty-two inches, likewise, subtract 50 points.

14. Do you have coronary artery disease? Subtract 100 points.
15. Do you have angina? Subtract 50 points if your angina is stable, 200 if it is not.
16. If you have congestive heart failure, subtract 200 points.
17. If your total cholesterol is over 200, subtract 50 points.
18. If your HDL cholesterol is over 55, add 100 points.
19. If your LDL cholesterol is over 150, subtract 50 points.
20. If your triglycerides are higher than 150, subtract 50 points if you are male, 100 if female. (Particularly in women, triglycerides are a more important predictor of heart disease than cholesterol is. If you don't know your cholesterol numbers, skip questions 17–20 and move on. But make a note to yourself to have your doctor prescribe a blood test. Knowing these numbers is vital.)
21. If you have had cancer that has responded well to treatment, subtract 100 points.
22. Are you on bio-identical hormone replacement therapy? If yes, pat yourself on the back and add 50 points to your total. (Although controversy swirls around the use of bio-identical hormones, we are convinced that they add function and vitality to a person's life, and that alone is sufficient to recommend them, assuming they are well managed. No studies have shown that estrogen, testosterone, or growth hormone increases cancer risk, but the remote possibility is continually batted around by medical authorities. Men in particular seem to benefit from having high levels of testosterone and growth hormone; the former confers the lowest risk of prostate cancer, and the latter confers longer telomeres.)
23. Do you experience memory loss of any kind? Subtract 100 points.
24. If you have been diagnosed with dementia, subtract 250 points.

25. Do you play bridge, or are you learning how to play a musical instrument or speak a new language? If any of these apply, add 100 points. (Challenging mental stimulation is associated with higher cognitive function, less memory loss and dementia, and longer life.)

26. Read the following sentence: A small white woolly bird ran sideways for one mile around a rubber track. Without looking again at the sentence, repeat ten times, "I want long telomeres," and then answer the following questions:
    a. What kind of animal was in the sentence?
    b. What did it look like?
    c. What action did it perform?
    d. How did it do this?
    e. Where did it go?
    f. How far did it go?
    Add 20 points to your total for each correct answer.

27. If you exercise less than three hours per week, subtract 100 points.

28. Do you exercise vigorously more than six hours per week? Add 200 points.

29. If 25 percent or more of your fitness routine is devoted to strength training, give yourself 100 points.

30. Do you take 3,000 milligrams or more of fish oil a day? Add 200 to your score. (Omega-3 fish oil is probably the most studied supplement. In our opinion, everyone should be on some form of omega-3 unless it is contraindicated.)

31. If you take at least one of the following antioxidants, add 100 points: ALA, CoQ_{10}, berry-derived anthocyanins, L-carnosine.

32. Are you happily married or in a happy long-term relationship? Add 200 points.

33. Do you belong to a social club or a house of worship that you participate in routinely? Add 200 points.

34. Do you have a pet that you care for and are bonded to? Add 100 points.

35. Do you have close friends you can talk to about anything? This is worth an additional 100 points.
36. Do you have a hobby that relaxes you and that you enjoy a lot? Add 100 points.
37. Do you meditate on a regular basis? Add 200 points.
38. What is your level of education? (Longevity correlates surprisingly well with education level. There are several possible reasons for this, including that more highly educated people tend to have higher incomes and thereby greater resources for maintaining their health.)
    a. If you finished high school or earned a GED and that's it, do not add or subtract any points.
    b. If you dropped out of high school and did not earn a GED, subtract 300 points.
    c. For every year of college you completed, add 100 points.
    d. For receiving a postgraduate degree of any kind, add 200 points.
39. What is your level of income?
    a. Less than $25,000 a year, subtract 200 points.
    b. Between $25,000 and $50,000, subtract 100 points only if you have dependents. If there are no dependents, subtract nothing.
    c. Between $50,000 and $100,000, add 100 points.
    d. Between $100,000 and $250,000 add 200 points.
    e. More than $250,000, add 300.
40. If you are male, subtract 100 points. If you are female, add 100. (Yes, studies show that, in general, women have longer telomeres than men of the same age.)
41. If you have age-related problems with your vision, such as macular degeneration, subtract 100 points.
42. If you have rheumatoid arthritis, subtract 200 points.
43. If you regularly use prescription drugs of any kind for any reason, subtract 100 points. (Besides the increased risk of side effects, there is absolutely no evidence that prescription

drugs have played a role in the slowly increasing longevity that humans are experiencing. There is even plenty of evidence that drugs and hospitals are correlated with declines in health and longevity.)

44. Do you routinely eat a nutritious breakfast? Add 200 points.

45. Do you often skip breakfast? Subtract 100 points.

46. Do you eat at least five servings of vegetables and two servings of fruits every day? Add 200 points.

47. Do you eat processed or smoked meat more than once a week? Subtract 250 points.

48. Do you drink fruit juices more than three times a week? Subtract 100 points. (You might as well eat a bowl of sugar.)

49. Do you frequently overeat and feel quite stuffed after a meal? If so, subtract 150 points.

50. If you eat fried foods more than twice a week, subtract 100 points.

51. Do you eat an optimal amount of protein on most days? Does the majority of this protein come from sources other than beef? If your answer is yes to both, add 150 points. ("Optimal" is the amount that does your body the most good, as opposed to "minimal," which is the amount you need to avoid being damaged. We can define optimal for a nonactive woman as 50 percent of her lean body weight in pounds × an additional 0.85 in grams, and 50 percent for a nonactive man [nonactive meaning no exercising]. For example, a nonactive woman at 130 pounds is about 70 percent lean body mass on average, so 62 pounds of lean body mass × .085 = about 50 grams of protein. The calculation for a man would be something like 180 pounds × 75 percent lean body mass × 0.85 rounded to about 75 grams of protein. For active men and women the increase in lean body mass [LBM] leads to an increase in protein demands and is reflected in these numbers: a 200-pound man with an LBM of 82 percent needs about 140 grams per day. For extreme

athletes of either sex, do not multiply by 0.85 and use the straight calculation LMB × weight = daily grams of protein. Define extremely active as more than ten hours of regular exercise per week.)

52. Do you mostly eat whole foods and seldom eat processed foods? Add 100 points.

53. Do you eat more than three eggs a week? If so, add 100 points.

54. If you drink three to six cups of green tea a day or take a green tea extract, add 100 points. (Green tea has been used as medicine in China for more than four thousand years. In more recent times, studies have established its effectiveness in inhibiting cancer cells and lowering total cholesterol, as well as improving the ratio of HDL to LDL cholesterol. A unique catechin (nutrient) in green tea, commonly abbreviated as EGCG, is not always fully used by the body. Consequently, you need to drink three to six cups a day or take an extract to get the full benefit.)

55. If you eat raw unprocessed nuts more than three times a week, add 50 points.

56. If you frequently eat salted nuts, subtract 50 points.

57. Do you consume an average of 30 grams of fiber per day from whole grains and/or fiber-rich beans, vegetables, and nuts? If so, add 200 points.

58. Do you consume olive oil every day? If you use olive oil for cooking, to put on salads, or perhaps even as a substitute for butter, add 100 points.

59. On an average day, if your diet includes at least two of these items—whole rather than nonfat or low-fat milk, cream, half-and-half, ice cream, real butter, cheese, or whole yogurt—subtract 150 points.

60. If you take a multivitamin every day, add 200 points.

61. Do you know what your vitamin D level is? If you do, give yourself 100 points for being health-conscious. (If your doctor has not tested you for this, ask him or her to do it now; the

vitamin D test is a simple blood test. If your doctor doesn't seem to know why this is important, get a new doctor!)

62. Do you take TA-65? Add 500 points.

63. How long can you hold your breath? (Test yourself to find out, if you don't know.) If you can't hold your breath longer than thirty seconds, subtract 200 points. If you can hold your breath longer than sixty seconds but less than ninety, add 150 points. If you can do ninety seconds or more, add 250 points. (There is a treadmill test you can take, called the VO2max test, that measures the maximum capacity of your body's ability to utilize oxygen during exercise. This, in turn, determines how physically fit you are, because lung capacity correlates with longevity and functional ability. The "how long can you hold your breath" test is not nearly as accurate in determining fitness; however, if you can hold your breath a relatively long time, your lungs are obviously fit.

64. Are you flexible enough to touch your toes while keeping your knees straight? Can you clasp your hands behind your back? If you can do both of these, add 200 points. If you can't, subtract 200 points.

65. Do you have sex with a partner or with yourself at least once a week? If so, add 200 points.

66. Without thinking, answer this question quickly and honestly: Is there a lot of stress in your life? If you said yes, subtract 250 points.

67. Generally speaking, on a day-to-day basis, are you happy? Add 200 points.

68. Generally speaking, on a day-to-day basis, are you unhappy? Subtract 100 points.

69. Do people perceive you as being hard to get along with? Subtract 100 points.

70. Do you see your primary-care doctor on a regular basis and take all of the tests he or she recommends? If so, add 300 points.

If you haven't been keeping a running total, add and subtract until you come up with your final number. Check this number on the scale below for an approximation of your average telomere length.

The Telomere Age Scorecard

Less than 5,000. Your telomere age is between eighty and one hundred years. We strongly suggest you get a telomere-length blood test as soon as possible.

5,001–6,000. Your telomere age is between sixty and seventy years. If you are younger than sixty years old, then you need to address the risk factors of aging now and start following the recommendations in this book. Consider telomere testing and, if you can afford it, TA-65.

6,001–7,000. Your telomere age is between forty-eight and sixty years. If this fits your age category, then you are aging normally. But is this what you want? If you want to live a longer, healthier life, it's time to get with the program!

7,001–8,000. Your telomere age is between thirty-five and forty-seven years. Now is a great time to modify any risk factors you have, exercise more, and eat better food. Your goal should be to slow down the deterioration of your telomeres so you can stay younger longer.

8,001 and higher. Eureka! Your telomere age is less than thirty-five, and you're doing great. Let's keep it there for the next fifty years.

Telomere Therapy

If your telomeres are short for your age, you can take TA-65, of course. But at up to $8,000 a year and not covered by most insurance policies, TA-65 is prohibitively expensive for most people, and its effect is not nearly as dramatic as new therapies will be in the near future.

The other option is to adopt the lifestyle, diet, and exercise changes we advocate. These won't turn on the telomerase enzyme, but they will dramatically reduce the rate of telomere shortening.

How It Works

Suppose your telomeres have aged two years more than your chronological age. If the average telomere loses forty base pairs a year and you can cut your losses to twenty base pairs per year, then in just four years you will have gained back the two years you lost. Keep it up for another four years and your telomeres will be two years younger than your chronological age. You will have successfully and completely reversed the situation.

Now let's go a step further. Imagine that it's fifteen years from now, and, as predicted by many anti-aging scientists and medical doctors, a drug therapy has been developed for turning on telomerase and reversing the age of humans. You're seventy-five years old with the typical blood vessels and organs of someone that age. How long will it take to reverse the damage done to them? Initially, you might guess that it would take as long to reverse the damage as it did to create it. After all, your telomeres required time to erode; it took different cells various amounts of time to fall prey to aging.

The good news is that resetting your telomeres is a more uniform process; they can all be reset within days of treatment. Although the resetting of the clocks could be fairly uniform and rapid, and although the time it requires could be independent of how long it took you and your cells to age, that still doesn't tell us how long it would be before we saw any change in *you*. Cells are one thing; you are another.

In your blood vessels, a single endothelial cell, whose job is to protect your vessel wall, previously unable to divide, would now almost immediately, perhaps within hours, be capable of division once again. It would then divide and provide better coverage of the inner wall. But how soon would the cholesterol deposits, macrophage cells (scavenger cells), and signs of inflammation recede, leaving the vessel open and smooth? Predicting this is a chancy affair, but most likely it would take between weeks and years.

Telomeres might be extended almost immediately, but clinical changes will take more time. Some improvements might never occur. We cannot expect to regain brain cells that have died, but we can expect to stop losing them to disease caused by aging cells.

Another positive aspect of telomere therapy is a lack of payback. We will not have to worry about reaching the age of 175 and then suddenly aging in a day or a year. Aging, whether it is the first time or after telomere therapy, works slowly. It takes time because your cells divide over decades. Telomere therapy won't change the speed of cellular aging; it will just change the number of years it takes for your body to grow old. Even in progeric children, for whom aging appears accelerated, the pace of the underlying process is the same as it is in normal people, but their cells start out old. Progeric children look old in only a few years because all of their telomeres are already shorter at birth.

In fact, if telomere therapy makes your telomeres long enough, it will take longer than it normally would before your body acts aged. Your cells will divide just as fast, and your telomeres will shorten just as fast, but if your clocks are wound further than they are in the normal young adult, it will take longer to become old.

Whether it takes decades or a century, repeat treatment will be necessary unless we lock the telomeres in place, which might further increase the risk of cancer. The conservative approach, at least initially, will probably simply be to periodically reextend the telomeres. Considering how long it currently takes your body to mature and how long it takes to age, you might expect to need treatment every few decades.

How It Will Feel

The process will probably go something like this: At age seventy-five you decide to try your first treatment. Let's say you have moderate arthritis. Stairs are uncomfortable to climb (moderate arthritis does not make it impossible to climb stairs), and getting out of bed in the morning is a chore. Your heart isn't what it once was, and you know it is a bit harder for you to do the kinds of things you did physically ten years ago. You tire walking over a block. It takes you a short period of time to catch your breath. You bruise a bit more easily and heal up more slowly than before. Even with all this, you consider yourself lucky, compared to many of your friends.

Nevertheless, you'd like more from life than shortness of breath, arthritis, and having to slow down more every year or so, so you make an appointment for telomere therapy. The first day you have a few blood tests and an examination. The second day you are given a pill; the nurse checks your blood pressure and watches you for half an hour before sending you home. But before you get home, the pill has already dissolved, and the active ingredient—a telomerase inducer—has gone into your bloodstream. Within an hour, some of your cells have begun to express telomerase. By nightfall, your cells are resetting their own telomeres.

A week later you're back. You haven't noticed any changes. Your blood pressure is the same, and so are your other tests. The doctor points out that the scrape on your arm has finally healed beautifully, and you notice that your liver spots are fading a bit and that your skin is firmer and healthier.

A month passes before your next visit, and you notice you can do more, feel less tired, and seem to have more stamina. A few of your friends are starting to ask what you are doing differently. Your arthritis didn't bother you as much the past two or three days, but the weather has been warmer. After the exam is over, you think about stopping at the library on the way home; you haven't had the energy to go there for a few years, but you've been eating better this week because your appetite has been better. Then you change your mind about the library and decide to go out to lunch.

Six months pass, and you've seen your doctor only once in that time. You stopped by to thank him after you played tennis for the first time in ten years. You and a friend have been traveling again, and surprise, surprise, you're even having sex again! When you're back home, there are so many things to do that you keep canceling the doctor's appointment. Maybe next month, if the bicycle you ordered comes, you might ride over and see what the doctor thinks of you—that is, if you can fit it in between tennis matches during the day and salsa lessons in the evening.

Although telomere therapy can help bring you back to the body of a younger man or woman with less fat, more muscle, and more energy, it will not prevent every aspect of aging. Telomere alteration can dramatically affect your health and most likely your life span, but it is not a total panacea. It won't make you invulnerable if you happen to walk by a car bomb at the wrong moment. It won't guarantee that you will never die of any disease you might otherwise acquire, and it won't make all of your other nontelomere-related genes any better than they are now.

The fact is that we all age differently, and certain genes take more of a pounding in some people's lives and bodies than in others' as a result of lifestyle and genetic characteristics. No one person gets exactly the same result from telomere therapy as another, but most seem to get a tremendous benefit that justifies the cost and the effort in their minds and the minds of their doctors.

Just because telomere therapy helps fight against the disease of aging we mention numerous times in this book, this doesn't mean you won't have one. It doesn't necessarily make it safer to eat foods high in cholesterol; it just makes a heart attack less likely. There will be every bit as much reason to exercise, to avoid saturated fats, to stop smoking, and to pursue the lifestyle habits we recommend in this book.

PART THREE

The Immortality
Edge Forever

6

The Immortality Edge
Forever Nutrition Plan

W e love food, and we want you to love food, too. There is significant science behind caloric restriction as a longevity tool, and we strongly suggest that as an accommodation to this tool you at least begin to reduce the amount of food you eat during any particular meal. The rule of thumb is to eat foods with fewer and more nutritious calories per bite. Overloading on calories puts a tremendous strain on your digestive system, which transfers all the way down to the cellular level, causing an increase in inflammation and oxidative stress—thereby accelerating the rate of telomere shortening. (For those who want to "cheat," the Life Extension Foundation offers a supplement, CR Mimetic Longevity Formula, that mimics caloric restriction. Go to www .LEF.org for more information.)

Trillions of cells in your body need good nutrition to avert potential damage and miscommunications, expel toxic substances, repair injured cells, prevent cells with damaged genes from reproducing, and keep you in good health. Too much nutrition at any one time, however, is like flooding an automobile motor with too much gasoline. The cells "gag" as they go into overload; they sputter and spew out free radicals, and the mitochondria lose their efficiency.

Just think back to your last really huge meal—maybe it was on Thanksgiving. How did you feel afterward? Were you energized? Ready to go out for a jog? Or did you feel tremendously tired and lethargic? Did you wish you had slowed down, eaten one less helping of mashed potatoes or skipped the chocolate cake?

Learning to eat less is not that hard to do. On the island of Okinawa, where there are by far more people over one hundred years old per capita than anywhere else in the world, people practice a philosophy of moderation in eating called *hara hachi bu*. The translation of this phrase is "eight parts out of ten," and it means that Okinawans stop eating when they feel about 80 percent full. As a consequence, their bodies form fewer free radicals during the process of metabolism. Indeed, studies of older Okinawans reveal consistently low blood levels of free radicals as well as impressively youthful clean arteries and low cholesterol.

At this point you may be wondering, "If I eat less at each meal, won't I be hungry during the rest of the day?" Our answer to this is that while we advocate eating less, we also advocate eating more often. Ours is a "never too hungry, never too full" strategy. Never skip breakfast, and instead of eating three large meals a day, eat five smaller ones—breakfast, lunch, dinner, and two snacks. You won't be overloading your cells, letting them run low before replenishing them. Instead you'll be providing your body (and your cells) with a more consistent steady flow of nutrition. This will also help you maintain a balanced blood sugar level, which is very important for losing weight or keeping you from gaining unwanted pounds. As one top scientist told us, "I would say that one is best off having more meals per day, especially meals at which relatively more carbohydrates (for example, fruit or potatoes) are *not* combined with meals with relatively more animal protein. Nuts and leafy stuff can probably go with either. This has to do with not mixing up insulin signaling."

An example of a one-day menu follows:

Carnivores

- Breakfast. A grain-free cereal (We'll explain why we suggest eating less or no grains in a bit. And www.lydiasorganics .com has terrific grain-free options) topped with a handful of berries. Add soy milk or almond milk. Black coffee or (preferably) black or green tea (with soy milk or almond milk only; skim or lowfat milk *if you must*).
- Mid-morning snack. ½ cup almonds or walnuts. Small amount of fruit.
- Lunch. Colorful salad topped with ½ cup grilled tofu, ½ chicken breast (not fried), wild salmon, or turkey. Water to drink plus tea or coffee.
- Evening meal: Steamed broccoli or similar green vegetable, yam or small baked potato, steak or roast pork. Water. Glass of red wine optional. No dessert except on special occasions.
- Night snack: Dark chocolate, small amount of fruit or nuts.

Vegetarians

- Breakfast. Same as above.
- Mid-morning snack: Same as above.
- Lunch: Substitute legumes for the chicken, wild salmon, or turkey.
- Evening meal. Grilled eggplant with side of baked tomatoes. Water. Glass of red wine optional. No dessert except on special occasions.
- Night snack: Same as above.

See our fourteen-day Immortality Edge Eating Plan at the end of this chapter.

So, as long as you don't eat much, it doesn't matter much what you eat? Of course it does!

You may have heard the saying "Food is medicine." This doesn't have anything to do with how it tastes, but rather with the beneficial impact it has on your body. The truth is that some food is medicine, some food is poison, and the rest is simply food. The nutritional secret to keeping your telomeres nice and long is to maintain a balance where the majority of food you eat is from the medicinal category and very little, if any, is from the poison category.

Knowing the Difference, Then, Is Key

You don't have to deny yourself the pleasure of exploring a vast universe of flavors and textures. You can learn to discern between foods that pack a tremendous amount of nutrition in a small volume (referred to as nutritional density) and others that yield much less. There is an endless variety of fresh, whole foods containing nutrients that energize your body and reinforce its ability to fight disease.

Top Twenty Telomere-Friendly Foods

1. *Blueberries.* The U.S. Department of Agriculture, in a comparison of one hundred foods, lists the blueberry as the best fruit source of antioxidants. Many studies indicate the blueberry's possible role in fighting such maladies as memory loss, high cholesterol, diabetes, and strokes. Eating blueberries improves blood flow, which keeps both your brain and your heart healthier. They contain a compound called pterostilbene, which has been shown to be very effective in reducing LDL cholesterol. It's no wonder that blueberries have such

an attraction as a health food: a mere half-cup serving has as much antioxidant power as five servings of other fruits and vegetables.

2. *Grapefruit*. There have been many studies over the years that associate eating grapefruit with weight reduction. Grapefruit (particularly red grapefruit) can also significantly decrease cholesterol and fight heart disease. Eating one red grapefruit a day for thirty days has been shown to reduce cholesterol by 15 percent and triglycerides by 17 percent. Separate the fruit from the skin before eating it—you'll get more fiber and more antioxidants. One concern is that grapefruit can have an accelerating and dangerous effect on some prescription drugs. Check the label on any prescription drugs you are taking before you add grapefruit to your diet.

3. *Almonds*. A true super food, almonds are a fantastic source of protein, fiber, and minerals including calcium, magnesium, iron, potassium, and zinc. They are high in vitamin E and contain monounsaturated fats, which can help to keep arteries supple. Stick to raw, unsalted almonds for maximum benefit.

4. *Apples*. Apples contain the phytonutrient quercetin, which prevents oxidation (damage) of LDL cholesterol, thus lowering the risk of damage to arteries and, in turn, the risk of heart disease. They also contain pectin, a soluble fiber that seems to be very effective in lowering levels of blood cholesterol.

5. *Avocados*. Pound for pound, avocados provide more heart healthy monounsaturated fat, fiber, vitamin E, folic acid, and potassium than any other fruit. They are the number one source of beta-sitosterol, a substance that can reduce total cholesterol, and lutein, an antioxidant that prevents cataracts and lowers the risk of prostate cancer.

6. *Beets*. Low in calories but packed full of nutrients, beets contain high levels of carotenoids and flavonoids that reduce

(continued)

(continued)

the oxidation of LDL cholesterol, protecting artery walls and reducing the risk of heart disease and stroke. They are one of the richest sources of folic acid. The silica in beetroot helps the body utilize calcium and boosts musculoskeletal health, reducing the risk of osteoporosis. Many people drink beetroot juice for its cleansing and detoxifying properties.

7. *Broccoli.* A "mega-longevity" food if there ever was one; researchers have found a wealth of healthy compounds in this vegetable, including two powerful anticancer substances, sulforaphane and indole-3-carbinol. According to research at Johns Hopkins University, sulforaphane destroys ingested carcinogenic compounds and kills the bacteria *Helicobacter pylori*, which cause stomach ulcers and greatly increase the risk of gastric cancers. Indole-3-carbinol metabolizes estrogen, potentially protecting against breast cancer. Broccoli is also a good source of beta-carotene and potassium. Many nutritionists suggest we eat broccoli three times a day.

8. *Sweet potatoes.* A sweet potato is nearly a meal in itself— full of protein, fiber, artery-protecting beta-carotene, blood pressure–controlling potassium, and antioxidant vitamins C and E. Unlike white potatoes, sweet potatoes won't send your blood sugar soaring.

9. *Garlic.* Numerous clinical trials have shown garlic to be an excellent cancer fighter—it has the ability to prevent development of cancers of the breast, colon, skin, prostate, stomach, and esophagus. Garlic stimulates the immune system by encouraging the growth of natural killer cells, which directly attack cancer cells. A study at the University of East London claims that garlic has the ability to not only kill many of the antibiotic-resistant strains of MRSA, the "hospital super bug," but is also able to destroy the newer super-super bugs that are resistant to the most powerful antibiotics used against MRSA.

10. *Olive oil.* Packed with healthy monounsaturated fat as well as antioxidants, olive oil is the main reason people who eat a Mediterranean-style diet have very few heart attacks and live longer, healthier lives.

11. *Oranges.* Research published by the *American Journal of Clinical Nutrition* has connected a higher intake of hesperetin, the main flavonoid in oranges, with lower rates of heart disease. Hesperetin helps protect against inflammation. Oranges are a rich source of pectin, which lowers cholesterol; potassium, which reduces blood pressure; and folic acid, which lowers levels of homocysteine.

12. *Wild salmon.* This is one of the best oily fishes, providing an excellent source of omega-3 fatty acids. Wild salmon has been linked with protection against heart disease, breast cancer and other cancers, and relief of autoimmune diseases such as rheumatoid arthritis and asthma. It's good for your brain, too. Even more exciting, high levels of omega-3s have been found to correlate with telomere length. The more omega-3s in your system, the longer your telomeres (we'll look at this in detail later on).

13. *Eggs.* Eggs are an excellent and inexpensive source of the highest quality protein. The myth about them being unfriendly to your cardiovascular system is just that, a myth. Eggs are also a good source of selenium, riboflavin, vitamin B_{12}, pantothenic acid, vitamin D, lutein, and zeaxanthin. These latter two nutraceuticals are carotenoids that protect your eyes from oxidative stress and ultraviolet light. And one more thing—eggs are the best source of choline, a neurotransmitter critical for brain function and health. Just one egg provides 23 percent of the recommended daily intake of choline.

14. *Tea.* Black, green, and now white teas have all been hailed for their antioxidant properties. According to epidemiological and animal evidence, green tea may inhibit breast, digestive,

(continued)

(continued)

and lung cancers. The polyphenols in green tea are powerful antioxidants (one hundred times as effective as vitamin C) and may protect cells from free-radical damage. A study published by the *Archives of Internal Medicine* found that people who drank two or more cups of green or black tea per day for ten years had higher bone density than those who didn't.

15. *Tomatoes.* Tomatoes contain high levels of lycopene, the consumption of which significantly reduces the risk of prostate, lung, and stomach cancers. It is best to cook your tomatoes before you eat them as this makes the lycopene more easily absorbable. Tomatoes also contain potassium, vitamin C, and beta-carotene, which is essential for the immune system and helps keep skin healthy.

16. *Meat.* We believe that meat may be very telomere friendly. With the exception of processed meats containing carcinogenic preservatives, lean meat represents an ideal way for anyone to get protein. Humans are adapted to eating meat genetically; we have a positive insulin-glucose response to lean meat. Meat proteins are anabolic, which helps the organism cope with physical stressors and survival and maintains the overall strength and power output that have been both indirectly and directly related to longevity. Meat also supplies needed iron, B_{12}, and zinc.

The degree to which people shorten their telomeres has more to do with oxidative stressors, which are the end result of physical and psychological stressors in the body. Meat's role in combating these stressors and helping the person remain strong and healthy suggests a positive role in keeping the telomeres longer.

The key point here, though, is to be sure you eat only organic, grass-fed meats. Bison is a perfect example of a "healthy meat." The Web site www.bisoncentral.com tells us

HEALTH: Bison are handled as little as possible. They spend their lives on grass, much as they always have, with very little time in the feedlot. They are not subjected to questionable drugs, chemicals or hormones. The members of the NBA feel so strongly about this that they have a resolution opposing the use of these substances in the production of Bison for meat.

NUTRITION: Research by Dr. M. Marchello at North Dakota State University has shown that the meat from Bison is a highly nutrient dense food because of the proportion of protein, fat, mineral, and fatty acids to its caloric value. Comparisons to other meat sources have also shown that Bison has a greater concentration of iron as well as some of the essential fatty acids necessary for human well being. *Readers' Digest* magazine has even listed bison as one of the five foods women should eat because of the high iron content.

17. *Beans.* All beans are loaded with energizing complex carbohydrates, calcium, iron, folic acid, B vitamins, zinc, potassium, and magnesium. They contain large amounts of both soluble and insoluble fiber, more than any other plant. The soluble fiber helps to reduce blood cholesterol levels and normalize blood sugar. Insoluble fiber helps regulate your bowel movements and may play a role in preventing colon cancer. Beans are cheap, too! (We include this food category for those who are vegetarian or who do not wish to embark on our Paleolithic Plan, explained later.)

18. *Sea vegetables.* No other type of food is as rich a source of minerals essential to maintaining and improving your health as sea vegetables, which we ignorant Westerners disparagingly refer to as seaweed. Because sea vegetables don't have roots like other plants, they must absorb nutrients from the ocean water. Dark sea vegetables, such as arame, wakame, hijiki, and certain varieties of kelp contain sodium alginate, which converts the heavy metals in your body into harmless sea salt, which

(continued)

(continued)

you subsequently expel when you urinate. Sea vegetables may account for the low rates of cancer in Japan. Sea vegetables also contain a high level of iodine, which aids in weight loss and can lower the amount of radioactive iodine absorbed by the thyroid by as much as 80 percent.

If you eat sushi, you are eating nori, which is a sea vegetable exceptionally high in protein and vitamin A, as well as other vitamins including vitamin K, iodine, and potassium. Dried sea vegetables can be added to cooked foods to add a salty flavor or eaten as a snack. Becoming familiar with sea vegetables and eating them every chance you get could add a few years to your life. "Seaweed" salad is delicious.

19. *Cabbage.* High in fiber, vitamin A, and all the usual minerals, cabbage stimulates the immune system, kills bacteria and viruses, inhibits the growth of cancerous cells, protects against tumors, helps control hormone levels, improves blood flow, and even boosts your sex drive. Eat enough and it will speed up the metabolism of estrogen and thereby reduce the risk of breast cancer and inhibit the growth of polyps in the colon. Studies have shown that eating cabbage once a week will reduce the risk of colon cancer by 60 percent. In its raw form, especially as a juice, cabbage contains ascorbigen, sometimes referred to as vitamin U, which heals and protects against stomach ulcers.

20. *Kale.* The richest of all leafy greens, kale might have even more medicinal qualities than cabbage. Like cabbage, kale helps regulate estrogen and wards off many forms of cancer, including breast cancer, bowel cancer, bladder cancer, prostate cancer, and lung cancer. It also protects against heart disease and helps regulate your blood pressure. The calcium in kale is more easily absorbed by the body than the calcium in milk—and kale has more of it. Kale is sometimes called the wonder food because eating enough of it protects against osteoporosis, arthritis, and bone loss.

Unfortunately, modern food technology has transformed slow-digesting grains into snack food made of pulverized starches that quickly raise blood sugar levels and promote insulin resistance and weight gain. Canned vegetables are overcooked and over-salted. Corn syrup is added to baked products and even canned fruit. The number of chemical additives on food labels is bewildering. Food that in its natural state would build you up has been turned into poison that tears you down.

Locally grown and seasonal organic fruits and vegetables are on top of our list of telomere-friendly foods. If you are lucky enough to have a farmers market nearby, we urge you to become a regular customer. Talk to the friendly people in the booths; many of them will be the actual farmers or producers, and they tend to be passionate and knowledgeable about the foods they are selling. You'll be amazed at what you'll learn about local growing conditions and techniques for raising produce without the use of pesticides, herbicides, or fungicides, or for humanely raising chickens and other animals without growth hormones and antibiotics.

Countless scientific studies have found a striking inverse relationship between consumption of fresh, whole fruits and vegetables and disease. The more daily servings you eat on average, the less likely you are to develop a chronic disease. Research into this phenomenon found that people who consume at least seven to ten servings a day get the most benefit. To accommodate that many servings, some of us have to rethink the concept that an animal protein (meat, fish, pork or poultry) has to be the most substantial part of our meals. It is very hard to eat a big piece of meat for lunch and again for dinner and still get enough veggies. Something has to give.

The American Institute for Cancer Research has reported, "Diets containing substantial and varied amounts of fruits and vegetables could prevent 20% or more of all cases of cancer." We believe you need to eat two to three servings a day of fruit and five to seven servings of vegetables. Before you freak out, let's first remember that we want you to eat five times a day, so if your two snacks each consist of one serving of fruits or veggies, you only have one or two fruits to go and five or six vegetables left. But to make it seem even more achievable, let's examine what a "serving" actually consists of.

A serving can't be quantified for all-purpose use, because it depends on the fruit or vegetable and how it's prepared. A serving of apple, for example, equals a medium-size apple, whereas a serving of cooked greens is only half a cup, compared to a serving of raw greens, which is a whole cup. It is not essential to know exactly what a serving is, but it is good to have an adequate approximation, so here's a chart:

Fruit or Vegetable	Serving Size
Apple, orange, banana, peach, or pear	1 medium
Baby carrots	6 to 7
Berries of all kinds	¾ cup
Broccoli	5 florets
Celery	2 to 3 stalks
Cooked vegetables	½ cup
Dried fruit	¼ cup
Grapes	17
Melon of all kinds	1 cup chopped
Orange or other fruit juice	½ cup
Raw fruit or vegetable	½ cup
Strawberries	6

Eating even bigger daily amounts of fruits and especially vegetables (they don't have the high sugar content of some fruits) is even more protective, so dig in. These foods won't make you fat, so you can pile your plate with two or three times the recommended amount of these servings. By doing so, you will boost your intake of antioxidants, vitamins, and minerals.

What about Vegetarians?

For the purposes of this book we offer a variety of eating options. As you will learn in the section on Paleolithic Planning, we believe that going on a hunter-gatherer eating plan will provide the optimum chance for extending lifespan. However, many people have strong feelings about eating meat and even eggs. Since fruits and vegetables are so good for you, shouldn't you just be a vegetarian? If you are a vegetarian, we don't want to do anything to dissuade you, and if you are considering it, go ahead, but not without taking a good hard look at Paleolithic Planning.

Most vegetarians, and especially vegans (people who don't eat meat or dairy) consume less saturated fat than carnivores do and thus have lower incidences of heart disease, obesity, and diabetes. Studies show that vegetarians are more insulin sensitive and can dispose of glucose better than meat eaters. A study of thirty thousand Seventh-Day Adventists found that vegetarians live about two years longer on average than meat eaters. Vegetarians who also eat nuts twice a week, exercise regularly and vigorously, maintain a healthy body weight, and never smoke live ten years longer.

While studies show vegetarians have fewer of the diseases listed previously, we believe that the fact that people are *conscious* about their lifestyle, that is, by being vegetarian, predisposes them to other healthy behaviors (exercise, yoga, meditation, nonsmoking) that added to their health and well-being, and that is why they may have scored high in those studies.

Do You Have to Eat a Fat, Juicy Steak to Get Enough Protein?

Made up of substances called amino acids, twenty-two of which are considered vital for your health, proteins are essential to the building, maintenance, and repair of your body tissue, such as skin, internal organs, and muscles. They are also major components of your immune system and hormones. Your body can make fourteen of these amino acids, but the other eight, known as essential amino acids, must be obtained from what you eat. Proteins are found in all types of food, but only meat, eggs, cheese, and other foods from animal sources contain complete proteins, meaning they provide the eight essential amino acids. For the Paleolithic Plan, however, cheese should be avoided.

Protein from vegetables, nuts, soy, and lean animal sources is ideal for our purpose of getting a lot of nutrition without overtaxing the body with too many calories. Eating protein actually boosts the chemical signals in your body that tell you, "You are not hungry," while squashing the "Eat now and eat a lot" signals. Be sure to seek out grass-fed beef, lamb, bison, and so forth and free-range chicken eggs only, if possible. You don't need to pollute your body with the hormones and other additives found in everyday meat and eggs.

The National Academy of Sciences (NAS) has set the daily Recommended Daily Allowance (RDA) of protein for males nineteen years old and older at 56 grams, and for females fourteen years old and older at 46 grams. Pregnant and lactating women require an additional 25 grams of protein per day for a total of 71 grams. For athletes who are doing strenuous aerobic exercises or intensive training we advocate extra protein.

Many nutritionists disregard all of this because their conventional theory is that the amount of protein a person needs is proportional to his or her weight. Their rule of thumb is that the number of grams of protein you need is your body weight (in pounds) multiplied by 0.37. So, if you tip the scales at 170 pounds, you need to eat 63 grams of protein a day ($170 \times 0.37 = 62.9$). To keep you from rummaging around for your calculator, here's a handy list to determine your baseline (nonexercising) protein needs based on your weight:

Body Weight	Proteins (Grams)
110	41
120	44
130	48

140	52
150	55
160	59
170	63
180	67
190	70
200	74
210	78
220	81
230	85
240	89

Now then, your average steak (T-bone, filet, porterhouse, and so forth) is about 25 percent protein. If you need 70 grams of protein a day, a 10-ounce steak will take care of all of this. The fact is that anyone who eats meat, poultry, or fish on a daily basis is probably getting enough protein, when you add all of the other sources, of which there are many. However, if you were to rely solely on spinach, which is fairly high in protein for a vegetable, you would need to eat 13 cups to get your 70-gram requirement—and we're talking boiled spinach, not raw.

Many vegetables contain protein, but just eating a variety of them as your only source will probably not add up to the minimum requirement. Add in some beans, lentils, and nuts, and things start adding up. Here's a list of protein-rich foods, excluding meat, poultry, and fish but including some dairy and bean/legume products for those who opt out of the Paleolithic Plan:

Food	Serving Size	Amount Protein
Soybeans	1 cup cooked	29 grams
Cheddar cheese	4 ounces	28 grams
Mozzarella cheese	4 ounces	26 grams
Tempeh	4 ounces	20 grams

(continued)

(continued)

Food	Serving Size	Amount Protein
Lentils	1 cup	17 grams
Cottage cheese	4 ounces	16 grams
Black beans	1 cup	15 grams
Kidney beans	1 cup	15 grams
Navy beans	1 cup	15 grams
Lima beans	1 cup	14 grams
Pinto beans	1 cup	14 grams
Yogurt	1 cup	12 grams
Peanuts	¼ cup	9.5 grams
Goat's milk	1 cup	9 grams
Tofu	4 ounces	9 grams
Pumpkin seeds	¼ cup	8.5 grams
Cow's milk	1 cup	8 grams
Almonds	¼ cup	7 grams
Oats, cooked	1 cup	6 grams
Egg	1	5 grams
Spinach	1 cup	5 grams
Asparagus	1 cup	4.5 grams
Broccoli	1 cup	4.5 grams
Brussels sprouts	1 cup	4 grams
Collard greens	1 cup	4 grams
Miso	1 ounce	4 grams
Mushrooms	5 ounces	4 grams
Mustard greens	1 cup	3 grams
Swiss chard	1 cup	3 grams
Green beans	1 cup	2.5 grams
Cauliflower	1 cup	2 grams
Romaine lettuce	2 cups	2 grams
Cabbage	1 cup	1.5 grams
Garlic	1 ounce	1.5 grams

Food	Serving Size	Amount Protein
Squash	1 cup	1.5 grams
Tomato	1	1.5 grams
Turnip greens	1 cup	1.5 grams

If you need 70 grams of protein and you're a vegetarian, you could easily get this amount by eating 4 ounces of cheddar cheese, 1 cup of black beans, a cup of yogurt, 2 eggs, and 1 serving of broccoli. If you're a vegan, it's a bit more complicated—1 cup of spinach, 4 ounces of tofu, 1 cup of lentils, 1 tomato, 1 cup of oatmeal, ¼ cup of almonds, 1 cup of squash, and 4 ounces of tempeh. Without the tempeh, however, you'd need to add about five other sources!

Paleolithic Planning: The Nutritional Holy Grail of Longevity?

We suggest that for optimum longevity, and if you are over forty, you convert to a Paleolithic diet. Why? Our good friend David Kekich, the founder of the Maximum Life Foundation, sums it up well:

> For millions of years, we subsisted on a hunter/gatherer diet. That means we ate what we could find and kill. Those diets were actually much more diverse than typical modern diets. Average life spans were quite short due to the harshness and dangers of everyday life. But contrary to popular belief, *maximum* life spans may have been much longer than we can hope to reach today.
>
> From 5,000 to 10,000 years ago, we entered the Agricultural Age. We started growing crops and domesticating animals. That's when we started eating grains and dairy products, and we were not adapted to them.
>
> We're not adapted now either, because 5,000 to 10,000 years is nothing on the human evolutionary scale. We are still adapted to the hunter/gatherer diet. We've been on it

for millions of years. We're also adapted to eating cooked meat and some vegetables, since we've been eating those for well over a million years.

By eliminating ALL grains and dairy products from your diet and by being physically active, you may be able to avoid most of the aging-related diseases. The sky is not the limit, but you could slow aging dramatically and may be able to add healthy active years to your life. Find out more by reading *Food and Western Disease* by Staffan Lindeberg.

If we look at a population from New Guinea, we see the benefits of the Paleolithic Plan. These people have no heart disease, stroke, dementia, diabetes, obesity, high blood pressure, or acne, and rarely such lifestyle conditions as cancer, arthritis, hip fractures, myopia, and tooth decay. The one-hundred-year-olds of this population look and act many decades younger.

David Kekich, in his book *Life Extension Express*, tells us,

Harmful foods that cause these diseases include modern staples such as grains, legumes, dairy, refined fats, sugar and salt. These were rarely available to hunter-gatherers, from whom we have inherited our genes, but they now provide the bulk of calories in most countries.

Grains and legumes destroy us in a number of ways. Plants contain toxic carbohydrate binding proteins called plant lectins that are designed to protect the plants against plant-eating animals. They poison predators to discourage them from eating the plants. The highest concentrations are found in grains, beans, potatoes and peanuts. Plant lectins are thought to be a major contributor to most modern diseases such as heart disease and cancer.

Since all plants contain lectins in varying concentrations, and since each contains its unique versions, you should eat a wide variety of fruits and vegetables in order to avoid concentrations of any one lectin high enough to harm you.

Grains and beans also contain protease inhibitors which inhibit protein-degrading enzymes in the digestive tract.

Phytic acid is found in grains and beans as well. It binds to minerals and trace metals and passes them through the digestive tract and keeps them from being absorbed.

Dairy is about as destructive. Casein, the major protein in milk, and lactose, the largest constituent in milk by weight next to water, are proven to be major aggravators and producers of atherosclerosis. Milk contributes to diabetes in most ethnic groups and contributes heavily to arthritis and other inflammatory conditions.

Do you see some of the ways grains, legumes and dairy kill us? Yet they are staples of recommended diets in the Western world.

Today, it's natural to die of a heart attack, which was almost unheard of before the Age of Agriculture. "Normal" blood pressure means you are at "normal" risk for a heart attack or stroke. Blood pressure and body weight should *not* increase with age. They only "normally" increase in sick populations. The majority of Westerners over sixty have *fully developed* atherosclerosis. So this again is "normal" for those of us with "normal" levels of blood pressure and serum lipids. Do you rejoice when your doctor says you are normal? The good news is, atherosclerosis is reversible in many cases by adopting a Palco lifestyle.

You can get all of the essential amino acids by eating a variety of vegetables, beans, whole grains, and nuts or by eating red meat, pork, chicken, or fish.

All things considered, the authors of this book opt to be Paleolithic Planners because we like meat, it is easier to get all of the complete protein you need, and we believe it to be the best dietary assurance for reaching a healthy and vital one hundred and beyond. This is the diet that is built into our genes. (It's not completely about denial, either, since yummy foods like cacao, avocados, and some honey have probably been part of our diet for millions of years.)

There is a very user-friendly and complete guide to this diet, and it is found in Dr. Loren Cordain's best-selling book *The Paleo Diet*. Loren explains the seven keys to the diet:

1. Eat a relatively high amount of animal protein.
2. Eat fewer carbohydrates than most modern diets, but eat good carbs from fruits and veggies.
3. Eat a large amount of fiber from nonstarchy fruits and veggies.
4. Eat a moderate amount of fat with more monounsaturated and polyunsaturated fats than saturated fats, and nearly equal amounts of omega-3 and omega-6 fats.
5. Eat foods with a high potassium content and a low sodium content, and do not add salt to your food.
6. Eat a diet with a net alkaline load.
7. Eat foods rich in plant phytochemicals, vitamins, minerals, and antioxidants, and do not eat grains, dairy, or legumes.

And here's the caveat, when it comes to eating meat, especially beef: we eat small portions and never more than once a day.

The Truth about Meat

Sarcopenia and dynopenia (age-related muscle loss and strength loss) are two independent problems that can be linked to poor quality and quantity protein intake, presumably from the shift in our diets away from meat and toward carbs. (Muscle strength in grip quadriceps and power generation are all directly or indirectly related to adequate protein intake and similarly to quality and quantity of life.)

Even studies linking red meat with lots of saturated fats (non–grass fed) to heart disease and stroke are actually poorly done, and while these studies are accepted by some politicians and others, they are not accepted by scientists. To date there has been no study linking red meat unequivocally to *any* disease process. Preserved and smoked meats may have negative health implications in large quantities, but even these findings are not clear-cut. Meat and protein cut hunger effectively and reduce insulin secretion and diabetes risk, as well as body weight. No studies linking high protein diets to kidney problems have ever been shown to have a real link in spite of recurrent appearances in the literature (unless, of course, you already have kidney problems). There are no studies linking meat to cancer that are scientifically accepted.

Paleo man took in more protein, more bulk, no sugar, more polyunsaturated and omega-3 fats, more micronutrients, much more potassium, no milk, no grains of any magnitude, and more water plus twice as many fruits and veggies as we do and had a low glycemic diet.

The bottom line? Meat of all kinds has not been shown to cause disease or decrease longevity. Neither has vegetarian eating been shown to improve longevity, it just changes the cause of death. Meat was and should be a major part of our diet and has numerous health benefits, not the least of which are appetite and obesity related.

Telomeres and the Paleolithic Diet

The last iteration of our genome with regard to the foods we eat seems to have taken place about fifty thousand years ago. At that time we were unquestionably small bands of hunter-gatherers who did not cultivate dairy animals or grains. History tells us these later "adaptations" did not take place until about ten thousand years ago.

We are still adapted genetically to the hunter-gatherer diet, also commonly known as the Paleolithic Diet, after this formative time of man's ascendance. Genetic anthropology has provided us with the gene structures to prove this. The last fifty thousand years have led to very little known genetic changes compared to our Paleolithic ancestors. Things like eye color and the occasional low-level persistence of the lactose gene into post-infancy do not change the fact that the bulk of what we eat now is actually not suitable for our genetic makeup. Dairy and grain products (which, according to a leading evolutionary biologist, can be tolerated by those under forty but not by those over, for maximum lifespan) provide the large mass of protein and carbohydrates that many cultures consume with potentially detrimental results to telomere length.

- Lactose intolerance is a common problem and ranges from mild discomfort to out-and-out "allergic"-type reactions with malabsorption of nutrients and leaky gut syndrome as a result.
- Grain intolerance, specifically to gluten, has become a modern-day mini-epidemic. As the sensitivity of testing procedures for these intolerances improves we may very well see that fully half of our population may have some variation of gluten sensitivity, ranging from minor to much more.

The telomere is pretty much the end arbiter of what we do to ourselves in all forms of stress, whether that stress comes from eating the wrong things, exposing ourselves to excess environmental toxins, sleep deprivation, too little or too much exercise, and so on. While specific dietary information and its relationship to telomere length is at this point extremely limited, the authors of this book predict the diet-telomere connection will truly be the "next big frontier" by which people can modify and improve their telomere length in a meaningful fashion.

Currently we know that fiber intake is positively associated with longer telomeres. We also know that excess inflammatory omega-6 fatty acids are bad for telomere length and that omega-3 fish oils are good.

We know that the complex web of insulin signaling and glucose excess directly affects inflammation, free-radical generation, and cell death. We know that vitamin D positively affects telomere length, as do tea-based catechins. But these are singular, piece-meal findings that do not equate to a specific diet pattern.

We strongly believe that the Paleolithic Diet is the most likely to provide this benefit, since our genetic makeup fits this type of diet to a tee. Studies have supported its positive effects on insulin signaling, oxidative stress, and endogenous acid load. We feel confident the end result will not only be longer telomeres but better health and potentially longer life.

Also, readers need not fear that when we talk about the Paleolithic Diet we are talking about eating raw meats and chicken, as other Paleolithic advocates have advised. Also, you can feel assured that cooked vegetables and tubers like yams are perfectly "legal" and healthy on this diet.

One other quick note: This diet is for those over forty, since adaptation drops drastically as we age and our modern diet is harmful, if not deadly, from that point on. It is not, however, recommended for children and could be counter-productive.

Fish

If it weren't for the plague of mercury contamination, fish would be by far the best choice over meat, pork, and poultry. The omega-3 in fish has been shown to play a significant role in maintaining a healthy cardiovascular system, preventing dementia, and keeping telomeres long. Scientific studies published in the *Journal of the American Medical Association* found that people with the highest levels of fish oil in their blood have the longest telomeres, and vice versa.

Sadly, in a recent U.S. Geological Survey, scientists found mercury contamination in every fish sampled in nearly three hundred streams across the United States. More than a quarter of these fish were found to contain mercury at levels exceeding the criterion for the protection of people who consume average amounts of fish. Other studies examining the fish in lakes and in the ocean have produced similar results.

Mercury in fish and the environment is largely due to the majority of our electricity being generated by coal-burning plants. A by-product of burning coal is the release of mercury into the atmosphere, which in turn is spread all across our planet by wind and subsequently dropped back to Earth whenever and wherever it rains. Bacteria in water convert mercury into a highly toxic form called methylmercury, which in turn finds its way into fish.

The larger the fish, the more likely it is to have a high level of methylmercury, simply because big fish eat little fish. As the National Resources Defense Council points out, large predatory fish, including tuna, swordfish, shark, and mackerel, can have mercury concentrations ten thousand times greater than those of their surrounding environment.

Compounding this problem is the fact that mercury bioaccumulates both in the bodies of fish and in humans. Once it is there, it is nearly impossible to get rid of, so every time you eat contaminated fish your mercury level rises. Infants and fetuses exposed to mercury can develop mental retardation, cerebral palsy, deafness, and even blindness. In adults, mercury poisoning has been linked to fertility problems, memory and vision loss, trouble with blood pressure regulation, extreme fatigue, and even neuromuscular dysfunction.

In an ideal world, fish would be the ideal food. It is high in protein and full of essential nutrients and healthy fats. This isn't the case, however, so if you are going to eat fish, you should eat it only once a week or so. And, most important, you need to be selective as to the type of fish you eat. One fish to avoid for sure is probably the most consumed of all—tuna. Forty percent of all the mercury contamination found in people in the United States comes from consumption of tuna. The worse possible form of tuna you can eat is sushi, which often has up to ten times more mercury than other tuna, followed by tuna steaks and canned tuna. It's enough to make you want to cry, right?

So what are the least dangerous fish to eat? We checked with the Monterey Aquarium (montereybayaquarium.org) in Monterey,

California, which publishes a series of pocket guides to the best fish to eat (and not eat) based on cleanliness and sustainability. Adding our own criterion, which is a high concentration of omega-3, we came up with the following list:

The Top Ten Telomere-Friendly Fish
1. Wild salmon from Alaska
2. Wild salmon from Washington State
3. Anchovies
4. Sardines
5. Pacific halibut
6. Striped bass
7. Black cod
8. Arctic char
9. Pacific cod
10. Petrale sole
11. U.S. farmed trout
12. Wild pollock from Alaska

Also good to eat, but containing less omega-3, are lobster, mussels, oysters, clams, scallops, and shrimp.

Chicken Can Be Healthy

The number one source of protein in the world, chicken is also the world's most versatile food. Roasted, broiled, grilled, or poached, and combined with a wide range of herbs and spices, there are at least a million ways to turn chicken to a tasty dish. Just 4 ounces of chicken (about half a breast) contains 34 grams of protein, more than 50 percent of what most people need. If it is not fried and is skinless, it has less than half the saturated fat of a similar portion of red meat.

Chicken is also a very good source of the B-vitamin niacin and the trace mineral selenium, both of which have cancer-protective characteristics. A 4-ounce serving of chicken provides 72 percent of the daily value for niacin and 40 percent of the daily value for selenium. Components of DNA require niacin, and a deficiency of niacin (as well as other B-complex vitamins) has been directly linked to genetic (DNA) damage. Selenium is an essential component of several major metabolic pathways, including thyroid hormone metabolism, antioxidant defense systems, and immune function. Accumulated evidence from prospective studies, intervention trials, and studies on animal models of cancer has suggested a strong inverse correlation between selenium intake and cancer incidence. Selenium has been shown to induce DNA repair and synthesis in damaged cells, to inhibit the proliferation of cancer cells, and to induce their apoptosis, the self-destruct sequence the body uses to eliminate worn out or abnormal cells.

But before you go on a chicken-eating binge, be aware that not all chicken is equal. If possible, purchase chicken that has been organically raised or that is free-range, since these methods of poultry raising are more humane and produce chickens that are both tastier and better for your health. Organically raised chickens have been fed an organically grown diet and have been raised without the use of hormones or antibiotics. Free-range chickens are allowed access to the outdoors as opposed to being confined to the henhouse. Small farms raise the best chickens, and while they cost more, they also taste better and are better for you.

Factory-farmed chickens, the kind sold by major labels at your grocery store and in fast-food restaurants, are typically raised in massive confined pens where they have to be fed a diet heavy in antibiotics to ward off infection. They are also given hormones to increase their weight, and that's not all. In recent years, a process called plumping has been common among unscrupulous chicken producers. Salt water, chicken stock, or seaweed extract, or some combination of these, is injected into chickens to increase their weight and price, which also radically increases sodium content by up to 700 percent. One 4-ounce serving of plumped chicken

Hidden Sources of Sodium

You probably know that eating too much salt is linked to high blood pressure. But are you aware of the high levels of sodium in processed foods and restaurant cuisine? The average American consumes 4,000 milligrams of salt per day—2,500 milligrams more than necessary. The American Medical Association says that any food with over 480 milligrams should be considered a high-sodium food and avoided. A Starbuck's cheese danish contains 750 milligrams, while a can of Campbell's Chunky Chicken Soup has 889 milligrams. Many of the dishes from Weight Watchers and Lean Cuisine have more than 600 milligrams of salt. The lesson is to avoid canned and pre-packaged food, and be careful what you eat when you go out.

has the same—or higher—sodium content as a typical large order of French fries.

How can you tell if a chicken has been plumped? Simple, just check the label for the words "contains up to 15% saltwater." Another way to tell is if the nutrition label says a 4-ounce serving contains more than 70 milligrams of sodium.

As long as you stick to the good stuff, you can eat chicken four or five times a week, never tire of it as long as you try different recipes and preparations, and get a high percentage of the protein you need with a minimal amount of saturated fat. This is why we like chicken!

Go for Healthy Pork

Sometimes referred to as "the other white meat," pork production has succumbed to the same type of industrial practices as beef and chicken production. The vast majority of pigs spend most of their lives standing in their own feces. Mostly confined indoors, many of them live in pens so small they can't even turn around. Sadly, pigs have been bred over the years to produce more meat in relation to the amount of feed they eat, and as a consequence, conventional pork has lost much of the flavor and nutritional value of old-fashioned farmed pork. It has become dry and tasteless.

If you can find a source of pork that is raised outdoors on smaller farms, then you should buy and enjoy it. Otherwise, forget about it. Also, as much as possible, forget about eating ham, bacon, and sausages, as their consumption is correlated with the rate of colon cancer and other cancers.

Eggs Are Great!

We love eggs. They are an important part of any Paleolithic Planner's diet. Eggs contain the highest quality of protein, called biological value protein (eggs 100 percent, milk 93 percent, beef 76 percent, fish 75 percent, and corn 72 percent). One average-size chicken egg has 5.5 grams of protein and only 68 calories.

Eggs are an excellent source of selenium, riboflavin, vitamin B_{12}, pantothenic acid, and vitamin D. They are also a good source of lutein and zeaxanthin, which are carotenoids that protect your eyes from oxidative stress and ultraviolet light, and, better yet, choline, which is a neurotransmitter critical for brain function and health. Just one egg provides 23 percent of the daily value for choline.

People whose diets supply the highest average dietary intake of choline from eggs or soybeans have levels of inflammatory markers at least 20 percent lower than people with the lowest average intakes, according to a study published in the *American Journal of Clinical Nutrition*. These markers include C-reactive protein, homocysteine, tumor necrosis factor alpha, and interleukin-6.

As you learned from chapter 1, inflammation quickens the pace of telomere shortening. It logically follows, then, that eating eggs on a regular basis is one more way to protect your telomeres and extend your lifespan.

You may wonder about cholesterol. Don't eggs contain a great deal of cholesterol that will clog your arteries and cause heart disease? The yolk in a single large egg does contain about 213 milligrams of cholesterol, but the absorption of this cholesterol by your body is minimized by another compound in eggs called lecithin. So, even though a good amount of cholesterol is consumed when an egg is eaten, most of it becomes unavailable for absorption and just passes through the body.

Researchers at the University of Connecticut have shown that eating three eggs a day does not raise heart disease risk factors (LDL cholesterol) in healthy older people. This is hugely important, because as many people age they eliminate eggs from their diets upon misguided advice from their doctors, and yet eggs are an affordable source of protein for people on fixed incomes.

Another study by the Food and Nutrition Database Research Center at Michigan State University of more than twenty-seven thousand subjects showed that the risk of cardiovascular disease in men and women did not increase if they ate more eggs. Surprisingly, it did the opposite. The people who ate eggs had lower overall cholesterol levels than those who didn't eat eggs at all. While men who ate two or three eggs per week had slightly lower levels than men who consumed four or more eggs per week, both had lower levels than those who abstained completely. In women, those who ate four or more eggs per week had the lowest cholesterol levels of all.

Assuming you get your eggs fresh from a good source, ideally local farmers who raise free-range chickens on organic feed, you can safely eat up to one dozen every week. Better yet, you can eat some of them raw in protein shakes. And you can forget about the ridiculous practice of just eating egg whites.

Fiber Is Crucial

Fiber cannot be digested and passes through your system virtually intact. Yet, getting enough fiber in your diet is an essential key to living a long, healthy life.

Eat enough fiber and you will reap many rewards, particularly improved intestinal function, which includes things we don't normally like to talk about (healthier stools, more frequent bowel movements, less constipation). But this is only the beginning. When fiber pulls water from your body into your intestines to keep things moving along it also tends to gather up nasty chemicals, some of which might be carcinogenic.

Fiber in your diet makes you digest food more slowly and tends to fill you up—eating lots of fiber will help you control your weight. People on a high-fiber diet can maintain their weight or even lose some weight while consuming more calories than people on a low-fiber diet. And fiber does wonders for your cardiovascular system by lowering cholesterol levels and reducing triglycerides and blood pressure. This adds up to a reduced risk of heart disease, heart attacks, and strokes. Fiber also increases insulin sensitivity and thereby helps prevent or control diabetes. It has also been shown to reduce the risk of colon cancer and breast cancer for women and prostate cancer for men.

In other words, the right amount of fiber in your diet facilitates the most efficient, least toxic digestive process, with the least amount of stress, which translates all the way down to a cellular level. Yes, fiber is good for telomere health.

Harvard University published a study on fiber showing that the risk of colon cancer is reduced by as much as 40 percent in people who eat the recommended amount of fiber. An earlier, 1992, study of 32,208 Seventh-Day Adventists found those who ate whole wheat bread versus white bread had an amazing 50 percent reduced risk of heart disease (whole wheat bread has three times the fiber of white bread). Other studies have shown that fiber reduces the risk of diabetes, intestinal problems and heart disease, and prostate and breast cancers. It is even good for your teeth—researchers from Canada who collected diet information from 34,000 men over a fourteen-year period discovered that the men who ate the most brown rice, dark breads, and other whole grains were 23 percent less likely to develop periodontitis than those who reported eating less than one daily serving of whole grains.

To get the full benefits of fiber, you need to eat about twice as much of it on a daily basis as the average person eats. The Institute of Medicine recommends that adult men under the age of fifty consume 38 grams of fiber. For adult women under fifty, the magic number is 25 grams. For men over fifty it is somewhat less: 30 grams. For women over fifty: 21 grams. To help you calculate how much this is, an ounce equals 28 grams, so 30 grams would only add up to 1.2 ounces. It's not much, but we are talking about the weight of the fiber, not the food itself.

Which foods have the most fiber? The answer is whole grains, beans, fruits, vegetables, nuts, and seeds. Whole wheat bread and pasta have three times as much fiber as bread and pasta made from white flour. Beans are loaded with fiber—just half a cup of kidney beans has 7.5 grams. Broccoli has more fiber than any other vegetable (½ cup = 4 grams). The following is a short list of other basic foods with good fiber content:

Foods with the Most Fiber Content

One cup of lentils	= 15.5 grams
One cup of black beans	= 15 grams
One cup of lima, pinto, or garbanzo beans	= 12.5 grams
Sweet potato with skin (medium)	= 12.5 grams
One cup of green peas	= 9 grams
One cup of wheat	= 8 grams
Raspberries (1 cup)	= 8 grams
Romaine lettuce (2 cups)	= 7.5 grams

Collard greens (boiled, 1 cup)	= 5 grams
Handful of almonds	= 4.5 grams
One cup of corn	= 4.5 grams
One cup of blueberries	= 4 grams
One cup of Brussels sprouts	= 4 grams
One cup of green beans	= 4 grams
Handful of peanuts	= 4 grams
One cup of oats	= 4 grams
One medium pear	= 4 grams
Spinach (1 cup cooked)	= 4 grams

Here's an example of how much fiber-rich food you would need to eat on an average day to get 30 grams of fiber:

½ cup beans	7 grams
One bowl of oatmeal	6 grams of fiber
One cup of broccoli	4 grams
Two slices of whole wheat bread	4 grams
One apple	3 grams
One orange	3 grams
½ cup of spinach	2 grams
Handful of walnuts	1.5 grams
Total	30.5 grams of fiber

Fiber does not provide vitamins, minerals, or calories—but when you eat it, you are eating whole grains, vegetables, fruits, and beans. Because of this, fiber-rich foods are rich in disease-preventing phytonutrients, including antioxidants and flavonoids.

Phytonutrient is a broad term covering a variety of active nutritional compounds found in plants that act on human cells and genes to reinforce our natural defenses against illness. Our knowledge of phytonutrients has exploded since they were discovered in test tube research into cancer-prevention in 1986—we now know they play a role in preventing all major diseases.

Antioxidants are a type of phytonutrient. The more familiar ones, including vitamins E and C, are colorless, while the less familiar ones, called flavonoids, are red, purple, orange, and other colors (the darker the color, the more potent the antioxidant). There are thousands of these little chemical substances. All are indirectly derived from photosynthesis, the process by which plants turn sunlight into simple sugars, complex carbohydrates, fats, and proteins.

Energy in plants and animals is driven by the exchange of electrons among molecules. As photosynthesis takes place, billions of electrons get all "excited" and zoom around like crazy. Most go where they are supposed to go, but a significant number stray off course, turning into "free radicals." Free radicals cause plants to get sick and die. Phytonutrients protect plants against free radicals by intercepting and sponging up electrons that have strayed off course.

In humans, free radicals damage cells and accelerate the progression of all age-related diseases. Since our bodies don't engage in photosynthesis we have no way of creating our own supply of phytonutrients so we must rely on getting them from our diet or supplements. The more fiber-rich grains, fruits, and vegetables we eat, the more disease resistant we become.

Good Carbs, Bad Carbs

Some carbohydrates ("bad" ones) are digested very rapidly and literally dump sugar into your bloodstream. You feel full and energetic for about an hour before your blood sugar level plummets, leaving you tired and hungry. Other carbohydrates ("good" ones) raise blood sugar slowly and steadily—you feel full longer and have continuous energy. An overwhelming amount of research shows that different carbohydrate-containing foods have dramatically different effects on glucose levels, and these differences have huge health implications.

There is a simple measure of carbohydrate quality called the glycemic index or G-I for short. Simple sugars (yes, sugars are carbohydrates) with the highest glycemic index score become glucose almost instantly. Starches like potatoes and rice and foods made from refined white flour including pasta, bread, bagels, and pastries have a high G-I. Beans and whole grains have a low G-I. Scientists have tested the glycemic index of hundreds of foods and carried out long-term studies on its potential to improve diabetes control, resolve the symptoms of metabolic syndrome, and reduce heart disease and even the onset of dementia.

Eating bad carbohydrates causes the glucose level of your blood to soar and your pancreas to produce a large spike of insulin. Insulin helps move the glucose out of your blood and into your cells. This system works well for a while but breaks down over time. High levels of insulin overshoot the mark, driving your glucose levels too low, which makes you crave more high G-I foods. This is also why you might find yourself tired in the middle of the morning if you had pancakes and syrup for breakfast.

Many people with poor eating habits get mid-morning or mid-afternoon blahs and often eat candy such as a chocolate bar or a

---

Do Not Drink Your Fruit

How many times have you been out for breakfast and the server automatically pours you a 12-ounce glass of orange juice? That glass may have the sugar and calories of up to 8 or more oranges, which adds up to 104 grams of pure sugar with over 520 calories, and no fiber! Meanwhile, a simple orange has 42 grams of fiber, 13 grams of sugar, and 65 calories. If you must drink juice, dilute it at least half with water.

few jellybeans. A vicious cycle ensues. Eating large amounts of high G-I foods leads to a quick spike of insulin, which leads to low glucose levels, making you hungry for more high G-I foods. Tragically, cells develop a lower sensitivity to insulin—often referred to as "insulin resistance"—and this can lead to a major health problem called metabolic syndrome, which in turn accelerates atherosclerosis and other aging processes. Or, worse, it leads to type II diabetes.

The glycemic index ranges from 0 to 100, with glucose (straight, no chasers) at the top. Carbohydrates with a high rating are ranked 70 and above; moderate is between 55 and 70; and low

The 10 Lowest G-I Fruits

1. Cherries (G-I value of 22).
2. Grapefruit (25). The low G-I of grapefruit may be due to its high acid content, which slows absorption by the stomach.
3. Pears (32).
4. Dried apricots (32). An excellent source of beta-carotene and high in potassium, this is a wonderful fruit for anyone worried about insulin sensitivity. Whole, raw apricots aren't that bad either, with a G-I of 57.
5. Apples (38).
6. Plums (39).
7. Apple juice (40). Take away the fiber, leave only the juice, and apples still have a low G-I. This is because the sugar in apples is mainly fructose. However, beware—apple juice is high in calories.
8. Oranges (42).
9. Peaches (42). Most of the sugar in peaches is sucrose (4.7 percent); fiber content and acidity account for this low value.
10. Grapes (46).

is below 55. Amazingly, there are a handful of foods, for example, dried dates from Australia (G-I 104), that rank higher than glucose. Paradoxically, even though fruit is loaded with sugar, most fruits have a low G-I. Fruit contains a fair amount of fiber, but not enough to explain the phenomenon. Fructose, the sugar in fruit, has a surprisingly low G-I value, measuring in with a 20.

No Matter What, the Amount Matters

When you eat carbohydrates, your blood glucose level rises and falls. The extent to which it rises and remains high is critical to your health and depends on two things: the nature of the carbohydrates (G-I value) and the amount. Just because you might be eating a carbohydrate with a low G-I value doesn't mean you can stuff yourself without consequences. And conversely, a small amount of a carb with a high G-I value isn't going to do much damage.

It doesn't take much brainpower to realize you are better off eating foods like nuts, beans, lentils, carrots, brown rice, and whole grains instead of white potatoes, white rice, pasta, candy, most ready-to-eat breakfast cereal, cakes, and white bread. As you become more familiar with what is healthy for your body and eat more of these foods you will discover they make you feel better.

You can create a vicious cycle in reverse. Eat moderate amounts of high-fiber carbohydrates and your digestive system will gradually release glucose into your blood causing a mild production of insulin, which will help maintain your insulin sensitivity. You'll have steady energy, and you won't be hungry for several hours. When you eat again, you won't feel so ravenous that you overeat.

The Bitter Truth about Sugar

The enemy of a healthy lifestyle, sugar appears in almost every prepackaged food in your grocery store—and it's often disguised. An estimated 73 million Americans have pre-diabetes or diabetes, making it the seventh leading cause of death overall. Eating sugar causes your body to increase its insulin production, and over time this causes insulin resistance, which in turn leads to diabetes. Studies have shown that sugar is actually an addictive drug. In addition to diabetes, sugar consumption leads to high blood pressure, high cholesterol, heart disease, weight gain and obesity, depression, allergies, and premature aging. The more sugar you eat, the more you can count *up* your age.

Everyone needs to get smart about how to detect sugar. The food poisoning—that is, processing—industry has come up with dozens of ways to add sugar without using the word *sugar* on the food labels. Ingredients such as fructose, corn syrup, barley malt, cane-juice crystals, caramel, dextran, dextrose, fruit juice, fruit juice concentrates, glucose, lactose, honey, molasses, maltose, malt syrup, and sucrose are nothing more than buzzwords for sugar.

All sugar is bad for you. Some nutritionists advise people to avoid refined sugar, such as that refined from cane or beet juice. The idea is that complex sugars, like those in honey or fruit juice, are natural and thus "better" for you. Perhaps they don't metabolize quite as fast, but once sugar is processed by your body its effects are pretty much the same.

Think of it this way: on a scale of 1 to 100, with 100 being the most harmful, refined sugar is 100 and honey is 97. And there is even one form of sugar that in our opinion is 100-plus, namely, high-fructose corn syrup. The processed-food industry loves this stuff, which they endearingly call HFCS. Made by converting cornstarch into glucose, it is cheaper than sugar, tastes sweeter than sugar, and when used in baked goods has a tendency to keep them moist.

High-fructose corn syrup is the most insidious of all sugars—it is the king—and can be found in a vast array of packaged foods and beverages. The introduction of HFCS into U.S. food in the early seventies and its rapid acceptance ramps up suspiciously close to the explosive growth of diabetes and obesity. If you look at the ingredients listed on labels you'll be shocked to find HFCS in ketchup, jams, crackers, high-end soft drinks, lunch meats, and many so-called natural or health foods. It is even in most mass-produced breads.

Amazingly, some HFCS-injected products are endorsed by the American Heart Association and carry its seal of approval logo with the message, "Meets American Heart Association food criteria for saturated fat and cholesterol for healthy people over age 2." Examples include Kellogg's Smart Start cereals and Kellogg's Nutri-Grain cereal bars.

Fructose is not just a substitute for sugar—it stimulates less insulin secretion and is excluded from entering brain cells. The latter means excessive fructose ingestion may result in blunting the body's ability to recognize when it is full. The result is that you tend to eat more.

While you can totally avoid HFCS by carefully reading labels, we want to be realistic. No one totally avoids sugar, and it would be hypocritical of us to expect you to do this. We admit it—we occasionally eat sugar. Don't spend the rest of your life not eating one more bite of ice cream or a small piece of chocolate cake. Simply cut back and be diligent, as your health and longevity depend on it.

Some Fats Are Good, Some Fats Are Not

Fat is bad, right? Well, not necessarily—some fats are actually good for you.

The main form of fat in our bodies is triglycerides. Your body can both store and manufacture these fats—the manufactured ones are mostly created out of carbohydrates, which is why eating pasta makes you fat.

Ninety-five percent of body fat is triglycerides; the other 5 percent is phospholipids and sterols. Phospholipids, found in practically every cell of the body, are essential to brain health. Although present in many foods, phospholipids are found in higher concentrations in soy, eggs, and the brain tissue of animals—which may provide a biochemical rationale for the folk wisdom that says eating brains makes one smarter. There are phospholipid supplements, but very few people have a deficiency and there is no known harm from having too much.

Sterols, however, are a different matter. The best known is cholesterol, a type of fat that attaches itself to protein molecules to be carried through your blood vessels.

As you have probably read a thousand times, there are two types of cholesterol, commonly called "bad" cholesterol and "good" cholesterol. The bad stuff is LDL, which stands for "low-density lipoprotein," while the good stuff is HDL, or "high-density lipoprotein." An excess of LDL can lead to the buildup of plaque in your arteries and actually kill you. Meanwhile, HDL fights back by carrying LDL to your liver, where it can be processed and excreted from your body.

Food does not contain either HDL or LDL—food contains various forms of triglycerides. Some triglycerides are good for you because they lower LDL, some may be good for you because they lower both LDL and HDL, while the rest are definitely really bad for you because they raise LDL.

All fats contain the same amount of calories. A gram of fat, whether it is a trans fat or a monounsaturated fat, has 9 calories. Meanwhile, a gram of protein or a gram of carbohydrates has only 4 calories (a gram of alcohol, which is also a carbohydrate, has 7). For this reason, it is a good idea to eat less fat—the conventional rule of thumb is fat shouldn't be more than 30 percent of your diet.

The Good Fats

Monounsaturated fats. Found in olive oil, grapeseed oil, hazelnuts, almonds, Brazil nuts, cashews, avocados, sesame seeds, and pumpkin seeds, these fats lower LDL cholesterol while leaving your HDL at the same level. The high consumption of olive oil in Mediterranean countries is one significant reason Mediterranean people have lower levels of heart disease.

Omega-3 fatty acids. This is the oil found in fish and in supplements, including cod liver oil. Your body utilizes omega-3s in the formation of cell walls, making them supple and flexible, which improves circulation and oxygen uptake. So omega-3 is important to good cardiovascular health. Consuming it regularly will lower your LDL cholesterol and total serum triglyceride levels. It can also reduce blood pressure.

The association between omega-3 and human health was first observed by scientists who found it puzzling that the Inuit (Eskimo) people living in Greenland suffer very little heart disease, rheumatoid arthritis, diabetes, and psoriasis, even though their diets are alarmingly high in fat from eating whale, seal, and salmon. Eventually the scientists figured it out—these foods are very high in a type of fat (omega-3 fatty acids), which must be really good for you.

The American Heart Association recommends we eat fish at least twice a week in order to maintain a desired amount of omega-3s in our systems. However, many people take supplements on a daily basis and/or eat fish more regularly. Omega-3s have been shown to reduce the inflammation associated with arthritis and psoriasis and may even reduce the odds of your developing dementia or Alzheimer's disease.

The two forms of omega-3 that are most beneficial are EPA (eicosapentaenoic acid) and DHA (docosahexaenoic acid).

The Not So Good Fats

Alpha-linolenic acid. This is actually an omega-3 found in flaxseed oil and in some other foods, which is converted by your body into EPA and DHA. The American Heart Association recommends eating ALA-rich foods including soybeans, canola, walnuts, and flaxseed; however, the extent to which your body converts ALA to EPA and DHA is limited.

Omega-6 fatty acids. Omega-6s are "essential" fatty acids, meaning your body cannot manufacture them and therefore they must be obtained from food. Dietary sources include cereals, whole grain breads, most vegetable oils, most baked goods, eggs, and poultry. There is supposed to be a balance between omega-6s and omega-3s—the ratio between the two should be 1:1 and no more than 4:1 (4 times as much omega-6). The average North American diet provides ten times the necessary amount of omega-6, making the average ratio 15:1. This imbalance contributes to the development of long-term diseases such as heart disease, cancer, asthma, arthritis, and depression and is one reason we recommend eating fish and taking an omega-3 supplement.

Researchers recently discovered that excessive levels of omega-6 acids accelerate the growth of human prostate tumors. The suspicion is that there is a link between the increase in prostate cancer rates and the increase in consumption of omega-6. Not all omega-6 fats are bad, however. One form, conjugated linoleic acid (CLA), which is found in grass-fed beef, appears to play a role in reducing overall cholesterol levels.

Polyunsaturated fats. Most vegetable oils, including safflower oil, canola oil, sunflower oil, and corn oil, are polyunsaturated fat. They tend to lower both LDL and HDL cholesterol levels; on this score they are definitely a mixed bag. Like monounsaturated fats, they are liquid at room temperature.

It is probably a huge mistake to use these oils for cooking. A toxin associated with heart disease and neurological disorders referred to as HNE forms in high amounts in these oils when they are cooked. HNE has been linked in numerous studies with all sorts of nasty things including heart disease, stroke, Parkinson's, Alzheimer's, Huntington's, liver ailments, and cancer.

These oils are fine for salads, although olive oil is better. Beware, polyunsaturated oils are found in most baked goods.

The Really Ugly Fats

Saturated fats. Solid at room temperature, saturated fats are considered by the "traditional" medical establishment to be the most detrimental of all the fats. Outside of smoking, excessive alcohol intake, and high-fructose corn syrup, they are public enemy number one.

Derived from animal products, saturated fats include butter, cheese, cream, and the fat in milk and meats. Eating these fats will raise your LDL cholesterol and serum triglyceride levels and as the saying goes, "harden your arteries." They are strongly correlated to heart disease. In recent years, this ironclad concept has gotten more than a bit rusty. First, there was Dr. Robert Atkins, who proved you could lose weight by eating a diet high in saturated fats but low in carbohydrates. Then along came the South Beach Diet, which says not all of the carbohydrates are bad for you, just the simple ones (as compared to complex carbs). And finally, there's the Women's Health Initiative's Low Fat Diet Study, which showed that saturated fats do raise your LDL levels, but not as much as previously thought.

Top Ten Tips for Eating Less Saturated Fat

1. Eat less dairy. Choose low-fat or nonfat milk and cheese. Try milk substitutes like soy milk or almond milk.
2. Trim all visible fat from meat before and after cooking.

3. Give up fried food.
4. Don't eat chicken skin or salmon skin.
5. Eat less meat.
6. Prepare soups and stews ahead of time so you can refrigerate them to let the fat harden. Remove the hardened fat and reheat.
7. Use corn tortillas—never flour tortillas.
8. Use olive oil instead of butter. Olive oil is great to cook with and great on toast.
9. Forget store-bought salad dressings—make your own vinaigrette by mixing extra-virgin olive oil with a delicious vinegar (balsamic, Champagne, raspberry, red wine—always checking the label to make sure no added sugar has been slipped in). Chop up some scallions or garlic for added flavor.
10. Learn to love fat-free, sugar-free, spicy condiments and sauces including salsa, Tabasco, picante, ginger, adobe, chipotle, and the many Asian hot sauces. Substitute these for the fat-laden stuff like ketchup and mayo.

Are saturated fats still bad? Well, a study of 447 dieters in Switzerland, where half of the participants were on a low-carbohydrate diet while the other half were on a low-fat diet, found that after a year, weight loss for each group was about the same. However, low-fat dieters experienced a drop of about 10 percent in their LDL and overall cholesterol levels, whereas the low-carb dieters experienced about a 10 percent increase.

Hydrogenated (and partially hydrogenated) fats—aka trans fats. Purely an invention of the processed food industry, these fats are polyunsaturated fats that have been turned from a liquid into a solid or semisolid form through a chemical process that should make you very leery: particles of nickel or copper are added to a polyunsaturated fat (usually corn oil) and heated to an extremely high temperature under pressure for up to eight hours while hydrogen gas is injected. The hydrogenation process destroys the essential fatty acids in polyunsaturated fat and replaces them with a deformity called trans-fatty acids. Because your body's digestive system is the result of thousands of years of evolution, guess what: it's not equipped to process these "Frankenfats." The result is an imbalance throughout your metabolism and fatty deposits in your arteries.

You probably think hydrogenated fats are a fairly new invention, but the first one was Crisco, which was introduced by Procter & Gamble in 1911. Today, hydrogenated and partially hydrogenated fats are found in almost every processed food from soups to chips, margarine, vegetable shortening, crackers, cookies, pastries, mixes of all kinds, even in some pasta and rice mixes. They can also be found in frozen foods, including pizza and pot pie, and of course, they are widely used in deep-fried foods, including French fries.

More than any other fats, hydrogenated, partially hydrogenated, and trans fats raise LDL levels, and there is little doubt they cause obesity, diabetes, and heart disease. You should simply avoid them at all costs.

A Fourteen-Day Immortality Edge Meal Plan

The following daily meal plans include options for coffee or tea. We include these because so many people are literally addicted to their morning or daily caffeine and this plan is *not* about deprivation and hardship, be it real or otherwise. Plus, studies show the positive effects of limited amounts of coffee and caffeine and also a wealth of evidence showing us that black or green tea has healthful benefits. Enjoy your stimulation in moderation! For those who take their coffee other than black, the best choices of "whiteners" are soy or almond milk for Paleos and skim milk for non-Paleos. To sweeten we suggest stevia as a first choice followed by a high-quality blend of agave (that has not been refined or had corn syrup added) followed by turbinado or raw sugar in small amounts.

We include fruit options here and there as snacks and desserts. Melons, other than watermelon, are a good choice because they have fiber and good water content and the sugar is not immediately released into your bloodstream. Plus, they were around when we were developing our Paleolithic genes and have been consumed for millions of years. The problem is that now we have to deal with the issue of diabetes, so we need to keep sugar consumption low, and watermelon is a sugary choice as fruit. A fantastic choice whenever we mention fruits are berries, especially blueberries and blackberries, which are both full of anthocyanidins, known to be potent antioxidants and to improve vascular health.

Dried fruits, when listed, should be unsulphured, not sulphured, because sulphur is not a good choice as a preservative.

We didn't have room to include a vegan diet, but if you are a vegan you should be able to adapt the vegetarian menu to suit your needs. We don't expect anyone to slavishly follow this, but we hope you'll at least try to create an eating style that more or less fits the pattern that we present.

During the course of these days you should drink at least 8 glasses of water and you can drink up to 4 cups of coffee and/or black tea. If you drink green tea, drink as much as you like. Just don't drink soda, even the kinds with artificial sweeteners. New research has found that the phosphates in soda speed up the aging process.

Finally, and toward our goal of allowing the yin and yang in our nutrition and social choices, we allow red or white wine with dinner for those who do occasionally drink and for those who have a social life that includes the occasional cocktail party. We've all read about the benefits of resveratrol, and many people use that as an alibi for drinking red wine. While resveratrol is a useful element in *very* high dosages, the amount in a glass or two of red wine is *not* going to keep you alive for 150 years. However, wine is allowed on our program. We have even created our own cocktail, called the Edge, which is permitted in moderation. It is based on the main ingredient of a tequila called Patron, which is made with only the highest quality Weber Blue agave from Jalisco, Mexico, and is grown in rich volcanic soil. It is to distilled spirits what free-range, grass-fed beef is to other meats.

We all want to live long, be healthy, and prosper, but what good is all that health if it's not also fun!

The Edge Cocktail (Featuring your Patrón tequila of choice and budget!)

2 ounces Patron tequila of choice (or other brand, but we recommend Patron)
2 ounces cranberry juice (sweetened), pomegranate juice (sweetened), or Acai
splash of 7-Up to taste
5–10 drops astragalus extract (to taste)
one fresh or frozen blackberry (several blueberries will work if blackberries are not available)
Mix and serve over ice to taste.

The Edge Ultra

Same as above except mix with champagne of choice rather than 7-Up.

One more note before we begin. We list, from time to time, "shakes" or "super-smoothies." By concentrating tons of phytonutrients and healthy ingredients into the body via a liquid snack or meal, you will go a long way toward setting your body up for longevity. These liquid meals can be used anytime you experience hunger pangs that might otherwise cause you to make "bad" food choices. Use them as needed to avoid falling off your program. We suggest that you invest in a blending machine that is up to the task of delivering all of the nutrition available in healthy fruits and vegetables. Vita-Mix has been around for decades and is a reliable, effective choice, although a tad pricey for many. Montel Williams, the talk show host and now healthy living advocate, is a follower of eating along Paleolithic lines (especially when it comes to lots of fresh blended fruits and vegetables and healthy meat choices). His HealthMaster "emulsifier" is a remarkable tool for living the longevity life and is priced below the Vita-Mix. Also, the HealthMaster comes with a full recipe booklet that makes creating healthy smoothies a breeze. (The HealthMaster is available at www.myhealthmaster.com and in select retail stores.)

Day 1

Breakfast: Breakfast shake (whey protein, soy milk, berries, raw egg, a small amount of sweetener if you must). Black coffee or black tea, if you can tolerate this, otherwise, add a small amount of milk or almond milk. Paleolithic Planners get out your almond milk with grain-free cereal or two eggs cooked as you prefer.

Midmorning snack: One medium-size apple, whole or sliced, with a small amount of cheese. Paleolithic Planners replace the cheese with a handful of raw organic almonds.

Lunch: Colorful tossed salad with peppers, onions, tomatoes, other vegetables of your choice, and a few raw sunflower or pumpkin seeds. No cheese. Use an olive oil and vinegar dressing or any dressing that doesn't have added sugar. One slice of whole-grain bread or a roll brushed with olive oil, optional. Grain-free crackers or bread for Paleolithic Planners. Eat as much salad as you want. Unsweetened iced tea, water, coffee, or hot tea.

Dinner: Chicken prepared any way you like, except fried. Braised greens (such as chard, mustard greens, beet tops, spinach). Brown rice or, for Paleolithic Planners, a baked yam or potato. Water. One or two glasses of red wine optional. Fruit compote if you really must have some dessert.

Night snack: Raw or toasted, but unsalted nuts: almonds, cashews, walnuts, Brazil nuts, chestnuts, or pecans, but no peanuts. Just one kind or a mixture. A large handful or ½ cup up to one cup if you are really hungry.

Vegetarian Option

Breakfast: Same as above.

Midmorning snack: Same as above.

Lunch: Same as above.

Dinner: Baked stuffed tomatoes (whole-wheat bread crumbs, chopped garlic, lots of fresh basil). Braised greens (such as chard, mustard greens, beet tops, spinach). Brown rice or a small amount of boiled potatoes. Water. One or two glasses of red wine optional. Fruit compote if you really must have some dessert.

Night snack: Same as above.

Day 2

Breakfast: Scrambled eggs cooked in olive oil with a pat of butter if you want, unless you are a dairy-free Paleolithic Planner. Whole-grain toast (a grain-free cracker for Paleolithic types) with almond butter. One medium-size orange or grapefruit. Black coffee or black tea, if you can tolerate this, otherwise, add a small amount of milk or almond milk.

Midmorning snack: Raw or lightly steamed veggies: carrot sticks, celery, broccoli, or cauliflower. Just one type or any combination. Eat as much as you want.

Lunch: Mexican lunch without the rice. Whole pinto or black beans, guacamole, salsa, handful of chips, preferably unsalted. Fish or chicken tacos with whole-grain, corn tortillas. Unsweetened iced tea, water, coffee, or hot tea. Paleos will have their lunch without the chips or tortillas.

Dinner: Vegetable soup or onion soup. Grilled or pan-fried lamb chop. Cooked cabbage or cooked cauliflower. Water. One or two glasses of wine, optional. If you must have dessert, try flan.

Night snack: One medium-size apple, whole or sliced, with a small amount of cheese. Paleos replace the cheese with a small handful of nuts.

Vegetarian Option

Breakfast: Same as above.

Midmorning snack: Same as above.

Lunch: Mexican lunch without the rice. Whole pinto or black beans, guacamole, salsa, a handful of chips, (preferably unsalted). Red pepper, carrot, and Serrano pepper tamales. Unsweetened iced tea, water, coffee, or hot tea.

Dinner: Escarole or another another type of green-vegetable frittata. Carrot salad or beet salad with unsweetened vinaigrette. Water. One or two glasses of red wine, optional. If you must have dessert, try poached pears with a small amount of syrup or ice cream.

Night snack: Same as above.

Day 3

Breakfast: Breakfast shake (whey protein, soy milk or plain yogurt, ½ banana, raw egg, a small amount of sweetener if you must). Paleos enjoy a grain-free bread with organic fruit jam or two eggs any style. Black coffee or black tea, if you can tolerate this, otherwise, add a small amount of milk or almond milk.

Midmorning snack: Raw or toasted, but unsalted nuts: almonds, cashews, walnuts, Brazil nuts, chestnuts, or pecans, but no peanuts. Just one kind or a mixture. A large handful or ½ cup up to one cup if you are really hungry.

Lunch: Colorful tossed salad with peppers, onions, tomatoes, other vegetables of your choice, and a few raw sunflower or pumpkin seeds. No cheese. Use an olive oil and vinegar dressing, a yogurt dressing, or any dressing that doesn't have added sugar. One slice of whole-grain bread or a roll brushed with olive oil optional, but not for Paleos. Eat as much salad as you want. Unsweetened iced tea, water, coffee, or hot tea.

Dinner: One six-ounce grilled, broiled, or pan-fried steak. Assorted grilled peppers and onions. Sautéed mushrooms. One slice of grilled garlic bread, optional, unless you are going Paleolithic. One or two glasses of red wine, optional. Fruit compote if you really must have some dessert.

Night snack: small amount of dark chocolate, with or without nuts.

Vegetarian Option

Breakfast: Same as above.

Midmorning snack: Same as above.

Lunch: Same as above.

Dinner: Vegetarian lasagna or eggplant parmesan and broccoli or green beans. One slice of garlic bread, optional. Water. One or two glasses of red wine, optional. No dessert.

Night snack: Same as above.

Day 4

Breakfast: Oatmeal with berries and ½ banana, topped with a tablespoon of plain yogurt, soy milk, or nonfat milk. Black coffee or black tea, if you can tolerate this, otherwise, add a small amount of milk or almond milk. Paleos can gorge on a fruit smoothie made with one cup of berries, an apple, almond milk, and vegetable protein powder (found at health food stores).

Midmorning snack: Raw or lightly steamed veggies: carrot sticks, celery, broccoli, or cauliflower. Just one type or any combination. Eat as much as you want.

Lunch: Niçoise salad using anchovies, not tuna, with tomatoes, green beans, red pepper, cucumber, hard-boiled eggs, fresh basil, and lettuce plus an olive oil, lemon-based, unsweetened vinaigrette. Whole-grain roll or bread optional, preferably with olive oil, not butter, but not for Paleos. Unsweetened iced tea, water, coffee, or hot tea.

Dinner: Your favorite pasta with tomato sauce, garlic, chopped fresh basil, and a small amount of cheese. (Paleos enjoy a lean grass-fed meat of some kind, grilled to your liking). Radicchio salad, grilled radicchio, or your choice of any other healthy salad. One slice of grilled bread with olive oil and garlic unless you are a Paleo, in which case you may have a cup or two of lighty steamed veggies of your choice. Water. One or two glasses of wine, optional. No dessert.

Night snack: One slice of melon (cantaloupe, honeydew, crenshaw, or Persian, but not watermelon). One thin slice of cheese on top or a small amount of cottage cheese, optional. Paleos have fruit only.

Vegetarian Option

Breakfast: Same as above.

Midmorning snack: Same as above.

Lunch: Mediterranean lunch. Choose from tabouleh salad, hummus, grape leaves, and babaghanoush. Go easy on the pita bread. Unsweetened iced tea, water, coffee, or hot tea.

Dinner: Same as above.

Night snack: Same as above.

Day 5

Breakfast: Sauté a small amount of garlic in a skillet using olive oil or coconut oil; a pat of butter is optional but not for Paleos. Use this to cook a two-egg or three-egg omelet. In a separate pan warm up a mixture of leftover vegetables, tomatoes, salsa, or whatever suits your fancy. Fold the mixture into the omelet or just pour it on top. Eat with whole-grain toast brushed with olive oil, unless you are a Paleo. Black coffee or black tea, if you can tolerate this, otherwise, add a small amount of milk or almond milk.

Midmorning snack: A small amount of dried fruit (such as apple, pear, or prunes).

Lunch: Colorful tossed salad with peppers, onions, tomatoes, other vegetables of your choice, and a few raw sunflower or pumpkin seeds. No cheese. Use an olive oil and vinegar dressing or any dressing that doesn't have added sugar. Non-Paleos may have a slice of whole-grain bread or a roll brushed with olive oil, optional. Eat as much salad as you want. Unsweetened iced tea, water, coffee, or hot tea.

Dinner: Chicken cacciatore over brown rice or whole-grain pasta. A mixture of braised greens. Garlic toast, optional. Water. One or two glasses of red wine, optional. Sorry, no dessert. Paleos enjoy a grilled free-range chicken breast with braised greens.

Night snack: Raw or toasted, but unsalted, nuts: almonds, cashews, walnuts, Brazil nuts, chestnuts, or pecans, but no peanuts. Just one kind or a mixture. A large handful or ½ cup up to one cup if you are really hungry.

Vegetarian Option

Breakfast: Same as above.

Midmorning snack: Small amount of dried fruit (such as apple, pear, or prunes).

Lunch: Same as above.

Dinner: Orecchiette with fava beans and cherry tomatoes, olive oil, and a small amount of chopped onions. Substitute your favorite pasta with veggies if you must. One slice of grilled bread with olive oil and garlic, optional. Water. One or two glasses of red wine, optional. If you have to have dessert, try a baked apple.

Night snack: Same as above.

Day 6

Breakfast: Whole-grain toast (one or two slices, grain-free option for Paleos) brushed with olive oil, topped with almond butter and, if you insist, a very small amount of honey or jam. One whole medium-size orange or grapefruit or a handful of blueberries or raspberries (with yogurt for non-Paleos). Black coffee or black tea, if you can tolerate this, otherwise, add a small amount of milk or almond milk (Paleos).

Midmorning snack: Raw or lightly steamed veggies: carrot sticks, celery, broccoli, or cauliflower. Just one type or any combination. Eat as much as you want.

Lunch: Mediterranean lunch. Choose from tabouleh salad, hummus, grape leaves, babaghanoush, and chicken kabob. Go easy on the pita bread and avoid it completely if you are a Paleo. Unsweetened iced tea, water, coffee, or hot tea.

Dinner: Chicken prepared any way you like, except fried. Braised greens (such as chard, mustard greens, beet tops, spinach). Brown rice (non-Paleos) or a small amount of boiled potatoes. Water. One or two glasses of red wine, optional. Fruit compote if you really must have some dessert.

Night snack: A small amount of dark chocolate, with or without nuts.

Vegetarian Option

Breakfast: Same as above.

Midmorning snack: Same as above.

Lunch: Mediterranean lunch. Choose from tabouleh salad, hummus, grape leaves, and babaghanoush. Go easy on the pita bread. Unsweetened iced tea, water, coffee, or hot tea.

Dinner: Brown rice risotto with shallots or fennel and a small amount of Parmesan cheese. Roasted asparagus with arugula and lemon vinaigrette. Water. One or two glasses of red wine, optional.

Night snack: Same as above.

Day 7

Breakfast: Breakfast shake (whey protein for non-Paleos, soy milk, berries, raw egg, a small amount of sweetener, if you must). Black coffee or black tea, if you can tolerate this, otherwise, add a small amount of milk or almond milk.

Midmorning snack: One medium-size apple, whole or sliced, with a small amount of cheese (non-Paleo).

Lunch: Egg salad sandwich on whole-grain bread with lettuce—hold the mayo! Hold the bread if you are a Paleo. Coleslaw or shaved fennel salad. Water, iced tea, coffee, or hot tea.

Dinner: Wild salmon, baked, grilled, or poached. Boiled artichokes to be dipped in olive oil. You choice of root vegetable. Water. One or two glasses of white or red wine, optional. Poached fruit or fruit compote for dessert.

Night snack: Raw or toasted, but unsalted, nuts: almonds, cashews, walnuts, Brazil nuts, chestnuts, or pecans, but no peanuts. Just one kind or a mixture. A large handful or ½ cup up to 1 cup if you are really hungry.

Vegetarian Option

Breakfast: Same as above.

Midmorning snack: Same as above.

Lunch: Same as above.

Dinner: Lentil stew with chickpeas and Swiss chard, or any combination of your choice. Whole-wheat bruschetta topped with tomato and basil or with roasted red peppers and goat cheese. Water. One or two glasses of red wine, optional. Poached fruit or fruit compote for dessert.

Night snack: Same as above.

Day 8

Breakfast: Scrambled eggs cooked in olive oil with a pat of butter if you want. Whole-grain toast (non-Paleos only) with almond butter. One medium-size orange or grapefruit. Black coffee or black tea, if you can tolerate this; otherwise, add a small amount of lowfat, soy, or almond milk.

Midmorning snack: Raw or lightly steamed veggies: carrot sticks, celery, broccoli, or cauliflower. Just one type or any combination. Eat as much as you want.

Lunch: Chicken salad over tossed green salad. Whole-grain roll or bread, optional, preferably with olive oil, not butter. Water. Iced tea, coffee, hot tea, optional.

Dinner: Grilled or pan-fried hamburger using grass-fed beef, turkey, or buffalo. Cornucopia of grilled vegetables, which may include peppers of all colors, eggplant, zucchini, squash, onions, mushrooms, and corn on the cob. Water. One or two glasses of red wine or one glass of beer, optional. Watermelon for dessert.

Night snack: A small amount of dark chocolate, with or without nuts.

Vegetarian Option

Breakfast: Same as above.

Midmorning snack: Same as above.

Lunch: A large butter lettuce and spinach salad with grapefruit and avocado. Water. Iced tea, coffee, or hot tea, optional.

Dinner: Grilled or pan-fried veggie burger. Whole-grain bun, optional. Cornucopia of grilled vegetables, which may include peppers of all colors, eggplant, zucchini, squash, onions, mushrooms, and corn on the cob. Water. One or two glasses of red wine or one glass of beer, optional. Watermelon for dessert.

Night snack: Same as above.

Day 9

Breakfast: Oatmeal with berries and ½ banana, topped with a tablespoon of plain yogurt, soy milk, or nonfat milk. Paleos can have a super-smoothie made by blending ½ banana, a cup of sunflower seeds soaked overnight in spring water, drained, and rinsed, an apple, a cup of almond milk, and some ice. Black coffee or black tea, if you can tolerate this; otherwise, add a small amount of milk or almond milk.

Midmorning snack: Raw or toasted, but unsalted, nuts: almonds, cashews, walnuts, Brazil nuts, chestnuts, or pecans, but no peanuts. Just one kind or a mixture. A large handful or ½ cup up to 1 cup if you are really hungry.

Lunch: Niçoise salad using anchovies, not tuna, with tomatoes, green beans, red pepper, cucumber, hard-boiled eggs, fresh basil and lettuce, plus an olive oil, lemon-based, unsweetened vinaigrette. Whole-grain roll or bread, optional for non-Paleos, preferably with olive oil, not butter. Unsweetened iced tea, water, coffee, or hot tea.

Dinner: Black bean or three-bean chili with ground turkey or grass-fed ground beef. Shaved carrot, fennel, or artichoke salad. Water. One or two glasses of red wine, optional.

Night snack: One slice of melon (cantaloupe, honeydew, crenshaw, or Persian, but not watermelon). One thin slice of cheese on top or a small amount of cottage cheese, optional for non-Paleos. Paleos may enjoy a grain-free cracker with fruit-only spread.

Vegetarian Option

Breakfast: Same as above.

Midmorning snack: Same as above.

Lunch: Belgian endive and watercress salad with roasted walnuts and a shallot vinaigrette. Whole-grain bread or roll, optional. Water. Iced tea, hot tea, or coffee, optional.

Dinner: Baked stuffed tomatoes (whole-wheat bread crumbs, chopped garlic, lots of fresh basil). Braised greens (such as chard, mustard greens, beet tops, spinach). Brown rice or small amount of boiled potatoes. Water. One or two glasses of red wine, optional. Fruit compote if you really must have some dessert.

Night snack: Same as above.

Day 10

Breakfast: Non-Paleos can have whole-grain toast (one or two slices) brushed with olive oil, topped with almond butter and a very small amount of honey or jam, optional. Paleos may enjoy two free-range eggs prepared any style. One whole medium-size orange or grapefruit or a handful of blueberries or raspberries (with yogurt for non-Paleos). Black coffee or black tea, if you can tolerate this, otherwise, add a small amount of milk or almond milk.

Midmorning snack: Raw or lightly steamed veggies: carrot sticks, celery, broccoli, or cauliflower. Just one type or any combination. Eat as much as you want.

Lunch: Colorful tossed salad with peppers, onions, tomatoes, other vegetables of your choice, and a few raw sunflower or pumpkin seeds. No cheese. Use an olive oil and vinegar dressing or any dressing that doesn't have added sugar. One slice of whole-grain bread or a roll brushed with olive oil, optional for non-Paleos. Eat as much salad as you want. Unsweetened iced tea, water, coffee, or hot tea.

Dinner: Red pepper soup. Grilled or pan-fried halibut, sole, or black cod (the fish that is the freshest). English peas cooked with cocktail onions. Water. One or two glasses of white wine, optional. Your once-a-month dish of your favorite ice cream for dessert, optional. Paleos can "cheat" with a fresh-fruit-only sorbet.

Night snack: One medium-size apple, whole or sliced, with a small amount of cheese. Paleos can have a handful of Brazil nuts.

Vegetarian Option

Breakfast: Same as above. Paleos can have same a above, except substitute an egg or super-smoothie. A super-smoothie consists of a mixture or fresh greens—kale, or spinach, for example—combined with ½ to one whole apple, coconut water or spring water, ½ avocado, and several ice cubes, if desired, blended together to taste in your regular blender, or one of the machines described at the beginning of this meal planning section.

Midmorning snack: Same as above.

Lunch: Same as above.

Dinner: Escarole or another type of green-vegetable frittata. Carrot salad or beet salad with unsweetened vinaigrette. Water. One or two glasses of red wine, optional. If you must have dessert, try poached pears with a small amount of syrup or ice cream.

Night snack: Same as above.

Day 11

Breakfast: Saute a small amount of garlic in a skillet using olive oil or coconut oil; a pat of butter is optional for non-Paleos. Use this to cook a two-egg or three-egg omelet. In a separate pan warm up a mixture of leftover vegetables, tomatoes, salsa, or whatever suits your fancy. Fold the mixture into the omelet or just pour it on top. Eat with whole-grain toast (grain-free for Paleos) brushed with olive oil. Black coffee or black tea, if you can tolerate this; otherwise, add a small amount of milk, almond milk, or soy milk).

Midmorning snack: One slice of melon (cantaloupe, honeydew, crenshaw, or Persian, but not watermelon). One thin slice of cheese on top or a small amount of cottage cheese optional for non-Paleos. Paleos may enjoy a mini-super-smoothie prepared by using only 1/3 of previously listed ingredients.

Lunch: A large Greek salad. Go easy on the feta cheese, and if you can, forget the pita bread. Paleos be sure to avoid both completely. Water. Iced tea, coffee, or hot tea, optional.

Dinner: One six-ounce grilled, broiled, or pan-fried steak. Assorted grilled peppers and onions. Sautéed mushrooms. One slice of grilled garlic bread optional for non-Paleos. One or two glasses of red wine, optional. Fruit compote if you really must have some dessert.

Night snack: Raw or toasted, but unsalted, nuts: almonds, cashews, walnuts, Brazil nuts, chestnuts, or pecans, but no peanuts. Just one kind or a mixture. A large handful or ½ cup up to one cup if you are really hungry.

Vegetarian Option

Breakfast: Same as above.

Midmorning snack: Same as above.

Lunch: Same as above.

Dinner: Vegetarian lasagna or eggplant parmigiana and broccoli or green beans. One slice of garlic bread, optional. Water. One or two glasses of red wine, optional. No dessert.

Night snack: Same as above.

Day 12

Breakfast: Breakfast shake (whey protein, soy milk, or plain yogurt, ½ banana, raw egg, small amount of sweetener, if you must). Paleos use almond milk only. Black coffee or black tea, if you can tolerate this; otherwise, add a small amount of milk or half-and-half.

Midmorning snack: A small amount of dried fruit (such as an apple, pear, or prunes).

Lunch: Colorful tossed salad with peppers, onions, tomatoes, other vegetables of your choice, and a few raw sunflower or pumpkin seeds. No cheese. Use an olive oil and vinegar dressing or any dressing that doesn't have added sugar. One slice of whole-grain bread or a roll brushed with olive oil, optional for non-Paleos. Eat as much salad as you want. Unsweetened iced tea, water, coffee, or hot tea.

Dinner: Olives, a small amount of cheese and rye crackers for an appetizer. Paleos may enjoy a grain-free cracker with olive tapenade. Slow-cooked chicken legs in a pot with an onion, garlic, and kale or chard. Water. One or two glasses of red wine, optional.

Night snack: Raw or lightly steamed veggies: carrot sticks, celery, broccoli, or cauliflower. Just one type or any combination. Eat as much as you want.

Vegetarian Option

Breakfast: Same as above.

Midmorning snack: Same as above.

Lunch: Same as above.

Dinner: Orecchiette with fava beans and cherry tomatoes, olive oil, and a small amount of chopped onion. Substitute your favorite pasta with veggies, if you must. One slice of grilled bread with olive oil and garlic, optional. Water. One or two glasses of red wine, optional. If you have to have dessert, try a baked apple.

Night snack: Same as above.

Day 13

Breakfast: Scrambled eggs cooked in olive oil with a pat of butter, if you want and if you are non-Paleo. Whole-grain toast (grain-free for Paleos) with almond butter. One medium-size orange or grapefruit. Black coffee or black tea, if you can tolerate this; otherwise, add a small amount of milk or half-and-half. (Soy or almond milk for Paleos.)

Midmorning snack: One slice of melon (cantaloupe, honey-dew, crenshaw, or Persian, but not watermelon). One thin slice of cheese on top or a small amount of cottage cheese, optional for non-Paleos. Mini-super-smoothie allowed for Paleos.

Lunch: Mexican lunch without the rice. Whole pinto or black beans, guacamole, salsa, a handful of chips (preferably unsalted). Fish or chicken tacos with whole-grain, corn tortillas. Paleos may have a grilled bison burger or other grass-fed meat burger with a mass of organic salad greens and veggies and balsamic vinegraitte dressing. Unsweetened iced tea, water, coffee, or hot tea.

Dinner: This is a great time, for both Paleos and non-Paleos, to have a liquid meal. In fact, eating early and eating light for the last meal of the day one or two nights a week is a great way to stay lean and healthy. Blend a nutrient-dense veggie smoothie by combining a protein powder (whey or soy for non-Paleos, veggie protein powder for Paleos) with a cut-up whole apple, a cup of water, ½ cup of broccoli, ½ cup of carrots, and ½ cup of any other leafy green vegetable you have on hand.

Night snack: A small amount of dark chocolate, with or without nuts.

Vegetarian Option

Breakfast: Same as above.

Midmorning snack: Same as above.

Lunch: Mexican lunch with brown rice. Whole pinto or black beans, guacamole, salsa, a handful of chips (preferably unsalted). Red pepper, carrot, and serrano pepper tamales. Unsweetened iced tea, water, coffee, or hot tea.

Dinner: A small tossed green salad. Eggplant gratin with a side of baked tomatoes. Water. One or two glasses of red wine, optional.

Night snack: Same as above.

Day 14

Breakfast: Breakfast shake (whey protein, soy milk, berries, raw egg, a small amount of sweetener, if you must). Paleos may enjoy a super-smoothie. Black coffee or black tea, if you can tolerate this, otherwise, add a small amount of milk, soy milk, or almond milk.

Midmorning snack: Raw or toasted, but unsalted, nuts: almonds, cashews, walnuts, Brazil nuts, chestnuts, or pecans, but no peanuts. Just one kind or a mixture. A large handful or ½ cup up to one cup if you are really hungry.

Lunch: Chicken salad over tossed green salad. Whole-grain roll or bread optional, preferably with olive oil, not butter. (Paleolithic option, as always, is a slice of grain-free bread.) Water. Iced tea, coffee, or hot tea, optional.

Dinner: Vegetable soup or onion soup. Grilled or pan-fried lamb chop. Cooked cabbage or cooked cauliflower. Water. One or two glasses of red or white wine or an Edge Cocktail, optional. If you must have dessert, try flan (non-Paleos) or a cup of fresh fruits or berries.

Night snack: Raw or lightly steamed veggies: carrot sticks, celery, broccoli, or cauliflower. Just one type or any combination. Eat as much as you want.

Vegetarian Option

Breakfast: Same as above.

Midmorning snack: Same as above.

Lunch: Tofu salad sandwich. Make tofu salad by mashing tofu with finely diced bell peppers, celery, carrots, scallions, fresh herbs, and low-fat mayonnaise. Chill for half an hour. Spread thickly on whole-grain bread. Add mustard to taste. Serve with stewed tomatoes. Water. Iced tea, coffee, hot tea, optional. Paleos can have one hard-boiled egg with freshly sliced tomatoes and other assorted vegetables. One slice of grain-free bread or several grain-free crackers.

Dinner: White bean and eggplant gratin with Italian plum tomatoes. Sautéed kale. Water. One or two glasses of red or white wine, or an Edge Cocktail, optional.

Night snack: Same as above.

7

The Immortality Edge
Forever Exercise Plan

There are four steps to our exercise plan. The first step is to develop a stretching routine. The second step is to pick the level of exercise that's appropriate for you. The third step is what we call the Six Weeks to Fitness Plan, and the fourth step is what we call the Fitness Forever Plan.

Step One: Develop a Five- to Ten-Minute Stretching Routine

Before you do any type of aerobic, anaerobic, or resistance exercise, you absolutely, positively need to stretch gently and progressively for five to ten minutes. By increasing circulation to your muscles, stretching will warm them up and help you to avoid injuries. It will also strengthen them. Furthermore, stretching will improve your balance, which some day could actually save your life, because thousands of older people die each year from injuries caused by falls.

Stretching is completely individual and should be tailored to your particular needs—your particular muscle structure and level of flexibility. There are hundreds of stretches and much information, online and otherwise, that illustrate the proper way to perform each stretch. When done correctly, stretching feels good. It is not stressful; it is peaceful, relaxing, and noncompetitive. The objective is to reduce muscle tension and promote freer movement, not to attain extreme flexibility, which can lead to over-stretching and injury.

The stretches you incorporate into your personal stretching routine can be either static, in which you hold a position without moving for a certain amount of time (we recommend thirty seconds and no bouncing) or dynamic, in which you move while stretching. Reaching toward your toes and holding this position is an example of a static stretch, whereas slowly moving your head in circles is dynamic. You can also do a combination of the two, but again progression and common sense is the key. Listen to your body and avoid anything that is painful.

Your stretching routine should include a minimum of seven basic stretches, one for each of the following areas of your body: neck, shoulders, lower back, hips, hamstrings, calf muscles, ankles, and feet. If you practice yoga, this will be a piece of cake. You can simply use a combination of the poses you already know to cover the basic stretches without much help from us. If you already routinely do stretches during the day and/or before exercising, just keep doing them.

If you're not already stretching and you need some help, here's a great beginner routine you can adapt for your own purposes:

Immortality Edge Seven Basic Stretches

1. *Neck rotation.* Drop your chin straight down and slowly make a circle with your head in one direction, then repeat in the opposite direction. Do this four or five times.

2. *Shoulder stretch*. With your elbow bent, hold your left arm shoulder-high. Grip the elbow with your right hand and gently pull it across your chest toward your opposite shoulder. Release and pull three or four times. Switch, with your left hand pulling on your right elbow.

3. *Windmill stretch*. In a standing position, spread your legs so that your feet are positioned just outside your shoulders. Hold your arms out straight. Keep a slight bend in the knees. Bend forward from the waist in a twisting motion so that your right hand touches your left foot. Straighten up and repeat so that your left hand touches your right foot. Repeat up to ten times on each leg.

4. *Calf and Achilles tendon*. Using your hands, lean into a wall, and put all of your weight on your right or left calf. Using your toes, slowly raise and lower your foot, stretching your calf back and forth as far as possible five or six times. Repeat with the other calf. Then try doing this with the weight on both calves.

5. *Forward bend*. In a sitting position, sit with your legs together and extended straight out, again with a slight bend in the knees. Slowly bend forward at the waist and grasp your feet, if you can. If you can't, grasp your ankles or your shins. Gently move the crown of your head toward your feet as far as you can without hurting your lower back or rounding your spine and hold for thirty seconds while breathing slowly and deeply. Repeat once or twice.

6. *Foot and ankle stretch*. In the same sitting position as above, raise one foot off the ground a few inches and make a circle with it counterclockwise and then clockwise, six times each. Slowly move your ankle back and forth as far as you can. Repeat six times. Bend and stretch your toes back and forth several times. Lower your foot back to the ground and repeat with the opposite foot.

7. *Quadriceps stretch*. Roll over and lie flat on your stomach. Raise your right leg by bending your knee and grasp your

right foot, ankle or shin with your right hand. Pull with your hand gently toward your head and hold the stretch for thirty seconds. Repeat with your left leg. Then try to do this exercise with both legs at the same time. If you feel pinching in your lower back, stop. Keeping the feet flexed will help protect the knees.

If you already have a stretching routine, move on to the next step. Otherwise, spend two or three days practicing and perfecting your stretches.

Step Two: Determine Your Fitness Level

The core of our Immortality Edge exercise program is a high-intensity, interval, anaerobic routine designed to build up the capacity of your lungs, strengthen your heart, and boost your levels of human growth hormone by as much as 1,000 percent—and to do all this with the minimum amount of wear and tear (stress) on your overall cardiovascular, muscular, and skeletal systems. If this program is done correctly, your telomeres will remain long, you'll age more slowly, and, with any luck, you'll be around long enough to take advantage of future medical advances that will allow you to live indefinitely.

To get started, you need to know which of the four levels of our program will suit you best (from "out of shape" to "athlete"). If you have not exercised for a long time, or if you are overweight or unable to climb a flight of stairs without getting out of breath, then you're most likely a level one. If you exercise, but perhaps not as often as you know you should, you're probably a level two. If you exercise on a regular basis, then you're most likely a level three, although if you're in great condition you could be a level four. Let's find out for sure.

Begin by choosing the type of cardiovascular exercise that suits you best. Outdoor choices including walking, running, biking, jumping rope, swimming, or sculling. Indoor choices include jogging in place or using a treadmill, a stationary bicycle, a stair climber, a rowing machine, an elliptical trainer, or a ladder climber. You need only one, but once you get started, you can switch from one to another on different days, if you want.

Once you're in your proper gym clothes or a bathing suit and you're outdoors, at the gym, or at the pool, first do the five- to ten-minute stretching routine you developed for yourself with the previous guidelines. Once you've stretched, start your activity slowly and warm up for five minutes. Stay relaxed and don't exceed an effort level of 50 percent. If you're jogging in place, jumping rope, or climbing, do it for a minute or so, stop, and repeat two or three times. If you're walking, pick a path with a slight to moderate uphill incline.

Now that your muscles are loose and warmed up, test yourself with a timing device to see if you can sustain an effort level of 80 to 90 percent for thirty seconds. If you are swimming in a pool that is fifty feet or longer, you can swim one length of the pool and not time yourself. If the pool is shorter, swim a lap.

When you are ready, say to yourself, "Ready, set, go!" and take off. If you find that you can't sustain this level of exertion for thirty seconds or you become exhausted, stop. Otherwise, continue the exercise at an easy, slow pace for ninety seconds and then repeat the thirty-second burst, again at 80 to 90 percent effort. Keep doing this until you are exhausted, up to eight times.

Determine your level of fitness from the following chart:

Immortality Edge Fitness Level

Level one. You can't sustain an 80 to 90 percent effort for thirty seconds, or you can do this but don't have the energy to try a second time. *Don't be discouraged.* The famous Canadian endocrinologist Hans Selye, who coined the word *stress*, demonstrated that our bodies can adapt to most stresses if we endure them in small doses over time. In other words, if you consistently make the effort without overtaxing your body, you'll steadily become fitter and stronger. It might take a few weeks, but at some point in the near future, you'll be amazed and pleased with your progress.

Level two. You can do two to four repetitions without killing yourself, but after that you really don't feel like trying another one. This indicates that you are moderately fit and ready to work toward getting into great shape.

Level three. You can do five to seven repetitions before you feel like collapsing in a heap and not moving for the next day or two. Congratulations, you're in great shape and ready to rock and roll for the next hundred years.

Level four. You do the eight repetitions and say to yourself, "No sweat." You're an athlete and ready to go 100 percent the next time. This program is going to move you to superstar status!

Step Three: The Six Weeks to Fitness Plan

If you already do some sort of weight training or resistance exercise, you should continue at least one or two days a week, working it into the following program. We want everyone to do some resistance work, but it can wait until the end of this step, which is a six-week program that will put you into a regular rhythm, steadily increase your body's production of growth hormone, and get your heart and lungs in shape to move on to more frequent and intense workouts.

Based on your fitness level and the type of cardiovascular exercise you prefer, follow the daily routines as much as you can in the following charts.

Level One

Week 1

MONDAY

5- to 10-minute stretching routine
5-minute cardio warm-up

30-second burst at 50% effort
90 seconds at a very slow pace without stopping
30-second burst at 60% effort
90 seconds at a very slow pace without stopping
End with a few more stretches

Total time: 19 minutes

TUESDAY

5- to 10-minute stretching routine
5 minutes cardio exercise at a slow pace, with an 80% burst the
    last 15 seconds
End with a few more stretches

Total time: 15 minutes

WEDNESDAY

Take a break but get some extra exercise by walking a bit more than
    usual or climbing some stairs you wouldn't otherwise climb.

THURSDAY

5- to 10-minute stretching routine
5-minute cardio warm-up
30-second burst at 60% effort
90 seconds at a very slow pace without stopping
30-second burst at 70% effort
90 seconds at a very slow pace without stopping
End with a few more stretches

Total time: 19 minutes

FRIDAY

5- to 10-minute stretching routine
7 minutes cardio exercise at a slow pace, with an 80% burst the
    last 15 seconds
End with a few more stretches

Total time: 17 minutes

SATURDAY

5- to 10-minute stretching routine
5-minute cardio warm-up
30-second burst at 60% effort
90 seconds at a very slow pace without stopping
30-second burst at 70% effort
90 seconds at a very slow pace without stopping
End with a few more stretches

Total time: 19 minutes

SUNDAY

Take a long leisurely walk and enjoy being outdoors. If it is
hot, go early in the morning. If it is cold, bundle up! Spend
a few moments thinking about how good you feel, having
completed your first week of the Immortality Edge exercise
program, and how you are looking forward to next week.

Week 2

MONDAY

5- to 10-minute stretching routine
5-minute cardio warm-up
30-second burst at 60% effort
90 seconds at a very slow pace without stopping
30-second burst at 70% effort
90 seconds at a very slow pace without stopping
End with a few more stretches

Total time: 19 minutes

TUESDAY

5- to 10-minute stretching routine
7 minutes cardio exercise at a slow pace, with an 80% burst the
last 15 seconds
End with a few more stretches

Total time: 17 minutes

WEDNESDAY

Take a break but get some extra exercise by walking a bit more than usual or climbing some stairs you wouldn't otherwise climb.

THURSDAY

5- to 10-minute stretching routine
5-minute cardio warm-up
30-second burst at 70% effort
90 seconds at a very slow pace without stopping
30-second burst at 80% effort
90 seconds at a very slow pace without stopping
End with a few more stretches

Total time: 19 minutes

FRIDAY

5- to 10-minute stretching routine
7 minutes cardio exercise at a slow pace, with an 80% burst the last 15 seconds
End with a few more stretches

Total time: 17 minutes

SATURDAY

5- to 10-minute stretching routine
5-minute cardio warm-up
30-second burst at 70% effort
90 seconds at a very slow pace without stopping
30-second burst at 80% effort
90 seconds at a very slow pace without stopping
End with a few more stretches

Total time: 19 minutes

SUNDAY

Take a long leisurely walk and enjoy being outdoors. If it is hot, go early in the morning. If it is cold, bundle up! Spend a few moments thinking about how good you feel, having completed another week of the Immortality Edge exercise program, and how you are looking forward to next week.

Weeks 3–4

Repeat week 2.

Weeks 5–6

MONDAY

5- to 10-minute stretching routine
5-minute cardio warm-up
30-second burst at 70% effort
90 seconds at a very slow pace without stopping
30-second burst at 90%, accelerating to 100% effort the last 10 seconds
90 seconds at a very slow pace without stopping
End with a few more stretches

Total time: 19 minutes

TUESDAY

5- to 10-minute stretching routine
7 minutes cardio exercise at a slow pace, with a 90% burst the last 15 seconds
End with a few more stretches

Total time: 17 minutes

WEDNESDAY

Take a break but get some extra exercise by walking a bit more than usual or climbing some stairs you wouldn't otherwise climb.

THURSDAY

5- to 10-minute stretching routine
5-minute cardio warm-up
30-second burst at 70% effort

90 seconds at a very slow pace without stopping

30-second burst at 90%, accelerating to 100% effort the last 10 seconds

90 seconds at a very slow pace without stopping

End with a few more stretches

Total time: 19 minutes

FRIDAY

5- to 10-minute stretching routine

7 minutes cardio exercise at a slow pace, with a 90% burst the last 15 seconds

End with a few more stretches

Total time: 17 minutes

SATURDAY

5- to 10-minute stretching routine

5-minute cardio warm-up

30-second burst at 70% effort

90 seconds at a very slow pace without stopping

30-second burst at 90%, accelerating to 100% effort the last 10 seconds

90 seconds at a very slow pace without stopping

End with a few more stretches

Total time: 19 minutes

SUNDAY

Take a long leisurely walk, jog, or bike ride and enjoy being outdoors. If it is hot, go early in the morning. If it is cold, bundle up! Spend a few moments thinking about how good you feel, having completed another week of the Immortality Edge exercise program, and how you are looking forward to next week.

Level Two

Week 1

Increase to three bursts.

MONDAY

> 5- to 10-minute stretching routine
> 5-minute cardio warm-up
> 30-second burst at 70% effort
> 90 seconds at a very slow pace without stopping
> 30-second burst at 80% effort
> 90 seconds at a very slow pace without stopping
> 30-second burst at 80% effort
> 90 seconds at a very slow pace without stopping
> End with a few more stretches
>
> Total time: 21 minutes

TUESDAY

> 5- to 10-minute stretching routine
> 5 minutes cardio exercise at a slow pace, with a 90% burst the
>   last 15 seconds
> End with a few more stretches
>
> Total time: 15 minutes

WEDNESDAY

> Take a break but get some extra exercise by walking a bit more
>   than usual or climbing some stairs you wouldn't otherwise
>   climb.

THURSDAY

> 5- to 10-minute stretching routine
> 5-minute cardio warm-up
> 30-second burst at 70% effort
> 90 seconds at a very slow pace without stopping
> 30-second burst at 80% effort
> 90 seconds at a very slow pace without stopping
> 30-second burst at 90% effort
> 90 seconds at a very slow pace without stopping
> End with a few more stretches
>
> Total time: 21 minutes

FRIDAY

5- to 10-minute stretching routine

7 minutes cardio exercise at a slow pace, with a 90% burst the last 15 seconds

End with a few more stretches

Total time: 17 minutes

SATURDAY

5- to 10-minute stretching routine

5-minute cardio warm-up

30-second burst at 70% effort

90 seconds at a very slow pace without stopping

30-second burst at 80% effort

90 seconds at a very slow pace without stopping

30-second burst at 90% effort

90 seconds at a very slow pace without stopping

End with a few more stretches

Total time: 21 minutes

SUNDAY

Take a long leisurely walk and enjoy being outdoors. If it is hot, go early in the morning. If it is cold, bundle up! Spend a few moments thinking about how good you feel, having completed your first week at level two of the Immortality Edge exercise program, and how you are looking forward to next week.

Week 2

MONDAY

5- to 10-minute stretching routine

5-minute cardio warm-up

30-second burst at 70% effort

90 seconds at a very slow pace without stopping

30-second burst at 80% effort

90 seconds at a very slow pace without stopping

30-second burst at 90% effort
90 seconds at a very slow pace without stopping
End with a few more stretches

Total time: 21 minutes

TUESDAY

5- to 10-minute stretching routine
7 minutes cardio exercise at a slow pace, with a 90% burst the
last 15 seconds
End with a few more stretches

Total time: 17 minutes

WEDNESDAY

Take a break but get some extra exercise by walking a bit more
than usual or climbing some stairs you wouldn't otherwise
climb.

THURSDAY

5- to 10-minute stretching routine
5-minute cardio warm-up
30-second burst at 80% effort
90 seconds at a very slow pace without stopping
30-second burst at 90% effort
90 seconds at a very slow pace without stopping
30-second burst at 90% effort
90 seconds at a very slow pace without stopping
End with a few more stretches

Total time: 21 minutes

FRIDAY

5- to 10-minute stretching routine
7 minutes cardio exercise at a slow pace, with a 90% burst the
last 15 seconds
End with a few more stretches

Total time: 17 minutes

SATURDAY

5- to 10-minute stretching routine
5-minute cardio warm-up
30-second burst at 80% effort
90 seconds at a very slow pace without stopping
30-second burst at 90% effort
90 seconds at a very slow pace without stopping
30-second burst at 90% effort
90 seconds at a very slow pace without stopping
End with a few more stretches

Total time: 21 minutes

SUNDAY

Take a long leisurely walk, jog, or bike ride and enjoy being outdoors. If it is hot, go early in the morning. If it is cold, bundle up! Spend a few moments thinking about how good you feel, having completed another week of the Immortality Edge exercise program, and how you are looking forward to next week.

Weeks 3–4
Repeat week 2.

Weeks 5–6
Increase to four bursts.

MONDAY

5- to 10-minute stretching routine
5-minute cardio warm-up
30-second burst at 80% effort
90 seconds at a very slow pace without stopping
30-second burst at 90% effort
90 seconds at a very slow pace without stopping
30-second burst at 90% effort
90 seconds at a very slow pace without stopping
30-second burst at 90% effort

90 seconds at a very slow pace without stopping
End with a few more stretches

Total time: 23 minutes

TUESDAY

5- to 10-minute stretching routine
7 minutes cardio at a slow pace, with a 100% burst the last 15
   seconds
End with a few more stretches

Total time: 17 minutes

WEDNESDAY

Take a break but get some extra exercise by walking a bit more than
   usual or climbing some stairs you wouldn't otherwise climb.

THURSDAY

5- to 10-minute stretching routine
5-minute cardio warm-up
30-second burst at 80% effort
90 seconds at a very slow pace without stopping
30-second burst at 90% effort
90 seconds at a very slow pace without stopping
30-second burst at 90% effort
90 seconds at a very slow pace without stopping
30-second burst at 90% effort
90 seconds at a very slow pace without stopping
End with a few more stretches

Total time: 23 minutes

FRIDAY

5- to 10-minute stretching routine
7 minutes cardio exercise at a slow pace, with a 100% burst the
   last 15 seconds
End with a few more stretches

Total time: 17 minutes

SATURDAY

   5- to 10-minute stretching routine
   5-minute cardio warm-up
   30-second burst at 80% effort
   90 seconds at a very slow pace without stopping
   30-second burst at 90% effort
   90 seconds at a very slow pace without stopping
   30-second burst at 90% effort
   90 seconds at a very slow pace without stopping
   30-second burst at 90% effort
   90 seconds at a very slow pace without stopping
   End with a few more stretches

   Total time: 23 minutes

SUNDAY

   Take a long leisurely walk, jog, or bike ride and enjoy being outdoors. If it is hot, go early in the morning. If it is cold, bundle
   up! Spend a few moments thinking about how good you feel,
   having completed another week of the Immortality Edge exercise program, and how you are looking forward to next week.

Level Three

Week 1
Increase to five bursts.

MONDAY

   5- to 10-minute stretching routine
   5-minute cardio warm-up
   30-second burst at 80% effort
   90 seconds at a very slow pace without stopping
   30-second burst at 90% effort
   90 seconds at a very slow pace without stopping
   30-second burst at 90% effort
   90 seconds at a very slow pace without stopping
   30-second burst at 90% effort

90 seconds at a very slow pace without stopping
30-second burst at 90% effort
90 seconds at a very slow pace without stopping
End with a few more stretches

Total time: 25 minutes

TUESDAY

5- to 10-minute stretching routine
10 minutes cardio exercise at a moderate to fast pace, with a 90% burst the last 30 seconds
End with a few more stretches.

Total time: 20 minutes

WEDNESDAY

Take a break but get some extra exercise by walking a bit more than usual or climbing some stairs you wouldn't otherwise climb.

THURSDAY

5- to 10-minute stretching routine
5-minute cardio warm-up
30-second burst at 80% effort
90 seconds at a very slow pace without stopping
30-second burst at 90% effort
90 seconds at a very slow pace without stopping
30-second burst at 90% effort
90 seconds at a very slow pace without stopping
30-second burst at 90% effort
90 seconds at a very slow pace without stopping
30-second burst at 90% effort
90 seconds at a very slow pace without stopping
End with a few more stretches

Total time: 25 minutes

FRIDAY

5- to 10-minute stretching routine

10 minutes cardio exercise at a moderate to fast pace, with a
90% burst the last 30 seconds

End with a few more stretches

Total time: 20 minutes

SATURDAY

5- to 10-minute stretching routine

5-minute cardio warm-up

30-second burst at 80% effort

90 seconds at a very slow pace without stopping

30-second burst at 90% effort

90 seconds at a very slow pace without stopping

30-second burst at 90% effort

90 seconds at a very slow pace without stopping

30-second burst at 90% effort

90 seconds at a very slow pace without stopping

30-second burst at 90% effort

90 seconds at a very slow pace without stopping

End with a few more stretches

Total time: 25 minutes

SUNDAY

Take a long leisurely walk, jog, or bike ride and enjoy being
outdoors. If it is hot, go early in the morning. If it is cold,
bundle up! Spend a few moments thinking about how good
you feel having completed your first week at level three of
the Immortality Edge exercise program, and how you are
looking forward to next week.

Week 2

Increase to six bursts.

MONDAY

5- to 10-minute stretching routine
5-minute cardio warm-up
30-second burst at 80% effort
90 seconds at a very slow pace without stopping
30-second burst at 90% effort
90 seconds at a very slow pace without stopping
30-second burst at 90% effort
90 seconds at a very slow pace without stopping
30-second burst at 90% effort
90 seconds at a very slow pace without stopping
30-second burst at 90% effort
90 seconds at a very slow pace without stopping
30-second burst at 90% effort
90 seconds at a very slow pace without stopping
End with a few more stretches

Total time: 27 minutes

TUESDAY

5- to 10-minute stretching routine
10 minutes cardio exercise at a moderate to fast pace, with a
   90% burst the last 30 seconds
End with a few more stretches

Total time: 20 minutes

WEDNESDAY

Take a break but get some extra exercise by walking a bit more
   than usual or climbing some stairs you wouldn't otherwise
   climb.

THURSDAY

5- to 10-minute stretching routine
5-minute cardio warm-up
30-second burst at 80% effort
90 seconds at a very slow pace without stopping

30-second burst at 90% effort
90 seconds at a very slow pace without stopping
30-second burst at 90% effort
90 seconds at a very slow pace without stopping
30-second burst at 90% effort
90 seconds at a very slow pace without stopping
30-second burst at 90% effort
90 seconds at a very slow pace without stopping
30-second burst at 90% effort
90 seconds at a very slow pace without stopping
End with a few more stretches

Total time: 27 minutes

FRIDAY

5- to 10-minute stretching routine
10 minutes cardio at a moderate to fast pace, with a 90% burst
   the last 30 seconds
End with a few more stretches

Total time: 20 minutes

SATURDAY

5- to 10-minute stretching routine
5-minute cardio warm-up
30-second burst at 80% effort
90 seconds at a very slow pace without stopping
30-second burst at 90% effort
90 seconds at a very slow pace without stopping
30-second burst at 90% effort
90 seconds at a very slow pace without stopping
30-second burst at 90% effort
90 seconds at a very slow pace without stopping
30-second burst at 90% effort
90 seconds at a very slow pace without stopping
30-second burst at 90% effort
90 seconds at a very slow pace without stopping

End with a few more stretches

Total time: 27 minutes

SUNDAY

Take a long leisurely walk, jog, or bike ride and enjoy being out-doors. If it is hot, go early in the morning. If it is cold, bundle up! Spend a few moments thinking about how good you feel, having completed another week on the Immortality Edge exercise program, and how you are looking forward to next week.

Weeks 3–4

Repeat week 2.

Weeks 5–6

Increase to seven bursts, if you can; otherwise, stay at six.

MONDAY

5- to 10-minute stretching routine
5-minute cardio warm-up
30-second burst at 80% effort
90 seconds at a very slow pace without stopping
30-second burst at 90% effort
90 seconds at a very slow pace without stopping
30-second burst at 90% effort
90 seconds at a very slow pace without stopping
30-second burst at 90% effort
90 seconds at a very slow pace without stopping
30-second burst at 90% effort
90 seconds at a very slow pace without stopping
30-second burst at 90% effort
90 seconds at a very slow pace without stopping
30-second burst at 90% effort
90 seconds at a very slow pace without stopping
End with a few more stretches

Total time: 29 minutes

TUESDAY

5- to 10-minute stretching routine
15 minutes cardio exercise at a moderate to fast pace, with a
    90% burst the last 30 seconds
End with a few more stretches

Total time: 25 minutes

WEDNESDAY

Take a break but get some extra exercise by walking a bit more than
    usual or climbing some stairs you wouldn't otherwise climb.

THURSDAY

5- to 10-minute stretching routine
5-minute cardio warm-up
30-second burst at 80% effort
90 seconds at a very slow pace without stopping
30-second burst at 90% effort
90 seconds at a very slow pace without stopping
30-second burst at 90% effort
90 seconds at a very slow pace without stopping
30-second burst at 90% effort
90 seconds at a very slow pace without stopping
30-second burst at 90% effort
90 seconds at a very slow pace without stopping
30-second burst at 90% effort
90 seconds at a very slow pace without stopping
30-second burst at 90% effort
90 seconds at a very slow pace without stopping
End with a few more stretches

Total time: 29 minutes

FRIDAY

5- to 10-minute stretching routine
15 minutes cardio exercise at a moderate to fast pace, with a
    90% burst the last 30 seconds

End with a few more stretches

Total time: 25 minutes

SATURDAY

5- to 10-minute stretching routine
5-minute cardio warm-up
30-second burst at 80% effort
90 seconds at a very slow pace without stopping
30-second burst at 90% effort
90 seconds at a very slow pace without stopping
30-second burst at 90% effort
90 seconds at a very slow pace without stopping
30-second burst at 90% effort
90 seconds at a very slow pace without stopping
30-second burst at 90% effort
90 seconds at a very slow pace without stopping
30-second burst at 100% effort
90 seconds at a very slow pace without stopping
30-second burst at 100% effort
90 seconds at a very slow pace without stopping
End with a few more stretches

Total time: 29 minutes

SUNDAY

Take a long leisurely walk, jog, or bike ride and enjoy being
outdoors. If it is hot, go early in the morning. If it is cold,
bundle up! Spend a few moments thinking about how good
you feel, having completed another week on the Immortality
Edge exercise program, and how you are looking forward to
next week.

Level Four

Week 1

If you have been able to continue past six bursts and wish to really
push your fitness level to the max, then increase to eight bursts.

MONDAY

5- to 10-minute stretching routine
5-minute cardio warm-up
30-second burst at 80% effort
90 seconds at a very slow pace without stopping
30-second burst at 90% effort
90 seconds at a very slow pace without stopping
30-second burst at 100% effort
30 seconds at a moderate pace
30-second burst at 100% effort
30 seconds at a moderate pace
30-second burst at 100% effort
30 seconds at a moderate pace
30-second burst at 100% effort
30 seconds at a moderate pace
30-second burst at 100% effort
30 seconds at a moderate pace
30-second burst at 100% effort
30 seconds at a moderate pace
End with a few more stretches

Total time: 20 minutes

TUESDAY

5- to 10-minute stretching routine
15 minutes cardio exercise at a fast pace, with a 100% burst the
  last 30 seconds
End with a few more stretches

Total time: 25 minutes

WEDNESDAY

Take a break but get some extra exercise by walking a bit
  more than usual or climbing some stairs you wouldn't otherwise climb.

THURSDAY

5- to 10-minute stretching routine
5-minute cardio warm-up
30-second burst at 80% effort
90 seconds at a very slow pace without stopping
30-second burst at 90% effort
90 seconds at a very slow pace without stopping
30-second burst at 100% effort
30 seconds at a moderate pace
30-second burst at 100% effort
30 seconds at a moderate pace
30-second burst at 100% effort
30 seconds at a moderate pace
30-second burst at 100% effort
30 seconds at a moderate pace
30-second burst at 100% effort
30 seconds at a moderate pace
30-second burst at 100% effort
30 seconds at a moderate pace
End with a few more stretches

Total time: 25 minutes

FRIDAY

5- to 10-minute stretching routine
15 minutes cardio exercise at a fast pace, with a 100% burst the
    last 30 seconds
End with a few more stretches

Total time: 25 minutes

SATURDAY

5- to 10-minute stretching routine
5-minute cardio warm-up
30-second burst at 80% effort
90 seconds at a very slow pace without stopping
30-second burst at 90% effort

90 seconds at a very slow pace without stopping
30-second burst at 100% effort
30 seconds at a moderate pace
30-second burst at 100% effort
30 seconds at a moderate pace
30-second burst at 100% effort
30 seconds at a moderate pace
30-second burst at 100% effort
30 seconds at a moderate pace
30-second burst at 100% effort
30 seconds at a moderate pace
30-second burst at 100% effort
30 seconds at a moderate pace
End with a few more stretches

Total time: 25 minutes

SUNDAY

Take a long leisurely walk, jog, or bike ride and enjoy being outdoors. If it is hot, go early in the morning. If it is cold, bundle up! Spend a few moments thinking about how good you feel, having completed your first week at level 4 of the Immortality Edge exercise program, and how you are looking forward to next week.

Week 2

MONDAY

5- to 10-minute stretching routine
5-minute cardio warm-up
30-second burst at 80% effort
90 seconds at a very slow pace without stopping
30-second burst at 90% effort
90 seconds at a very slow pace without stopping
30-second burst at 100% effort
30 seconds at a moderate pace
30-second burst at 100% effort

30 seconds at a moderate pace
30-second burst at 100% effort
30 seconds at a moderate pace
30-second burst at 100% effort
30 seconds at a moderate pace
30-second burst at 100% effort
30 seconds at a moderate pace
30-second burst at 100% effort
30 seconds at a moderate pace
End with a few more stretches

Total time: 25 minutes

TUESDAY

5- to 10-minute stretching routine
20 minutes cardio exercise at a fast pace, with a 100% burst the
    last 30 seconds
End with a few more stretches

Total time: 30 minutes

WEDNESDAY

If you know how to do resistance training, spend an hour doing
    this.

THURSDAY

5- to 10-minute stretching routine
5-minute cardio warm-up
30-second burst at 80% effort
90 seconds at a very slow pace without stopping
30-second burst at 90% effort
90 seconds at a very slow pace without stopping
30-second burst at 100% effort
30 seconds at a moderate pace
30-second burst at 100% effort
30 seconds at a moderate pace
30-second burst at 100% effort

30 seconds at a moderate pace
30-second burst at 100% effort
30 seconds at a moderate pace
30-second burst at 100% effort
30 seconds at a moderate pace
30-second burst at 100% effort
30 seconds at a moderate pace
End with a few more stretches

Total time: 25 minutes

FRIDAY

5- to 10-minute stretching routine
10 minutes cardio exercise at a moderate to fast pace, with a
    90% burst the last 30 seconds
End with a few more stretches

Total time: 20 minutes

SATURDAY

5- to 10-minute stretching routine
5-minute cardio warm-up
30-second burst at 80% effort
90 seconds at a very slow pace without stopping
30-second burst at 90% effort
90 seconds at a very slow pace without stopping
30-second burst at 90% effort
90 seconds at a very slow pace without stopping
30-second burst at 90% effort
90 seconds at a very slow pace without stopping
30-second burst at 90% effort
90 seconds at a very slow pace without stopping
30-second burst at 90% effort
90 seconds at a very slow pace without stopping
End with a few more stretches

Total time: 27 minutes

SUNDAY

> Take a long leisurely walk, jog, or bike ride and enjoy being outdoors. If it is hot, go early in the morning. If it is cold, bundle up! Spend a few moments thinking about how good you feel, having completed another week of the Immortality Edge exercise program, and how you are looking forward to next week.

Weeks 3–6
> Repeat week 2.

Step Four: Incorporate Resistance Training into Your Routine

As we mentioned previously, you're never too old to pump iron. In fact, the older you become, the more important it is that you practice some form of resistance training, because otherwise you will start to lose bone density and could become in danger of getting osteoporosis. Contrary to conventional wisdom, osteoporosis is not a disease that strikes only elderly, skinny women who smoke. More than three hundred thousand men in the United States suffer an osteoporotic fracture each year.

Exercise—and, in particular, weight-bearing exercise—is instrumental to the creation of new bone tissue. The cells within the bones sense the stress of this type of exercise and respond by making the bones stronger and denser. Walking, dancing, jogging, stair climbing, rowing, tennis, and hiking are all weight-bearing activities, but none is as effective as resistance training. No matter how old or out of shape you are, resistance training will make you stronger and improve your bone health.

Resistance exercise is any exercise in which the muscles contract against an external resistance with the objective of increasing strength, tone, mass, and muscular endurance. The resistance can come from dumbbells, weight machines, elastic tubing or bands, cables, cinder blocks, cans of soup, our own body weight, or any other object that forces your muscles to contract.

Just as you created a stretching routine in step one, now is the time to create your very own resistance routine. With this addition, you'll have a complete exercise program: one that increases your endurance, boosts your cardiovascular system, enlarges your lung capacity, strengthens your muscles, increases your bone density, and floods your body with growth hormone without overloading it with cortisol, the stress hormone. This will put the brakes on telomere shortening. You'll feel great and not only look younger than your chronological age, you'll actually *be* younger, in a biological sense.

The first decision you need to make is what kind of resistance training you want to do. If you belong to a gym, you probably have the option of using free weights or weight machines. Some gyms also have machines that use cables, and some even have elastic bands. You can focus on just one of these choices, or you can use a combination.

The most important point about resistance training is that you've got to get it right. It is absolutely vital to do resistance exercises correctly. If you're not already pumping iron and don't know how to do the exercises safely and properly, we strongly advise you to get some help: take a weight-training class or hire a trainer at your gym to give you individual instruction. Otherwise, you may be risking serious injury, which could set you back for a very long time. If these options aren't available, at least find a knowledgeable friend to help you or buy an instructional video.

Your resistance-training routine should include at least one exercise for each of the seven areas of your body: shoulders, chest, back, biceps, triceps, abdominals (core), and lower body. There are dozens of choices within each of these groups. If you're not already into resistance training and you don't have access to a trainer who can help you create your own routine, here's one you can follow:

Immortality Edge Seven Basic Resistance Training Exercises

1. *Push-ups.* The push-up is a tremendously versatile exercise that engages nearly every muscle in the body, with an emphasis on the chest and the arms. Also, you can do push-ups everywhere, so they are a great exercise when you're traveling.

    On your hands and knees, place your hands shoulder-width apart. Stretch your legs back and come onto your toes. Bend your arms and lower your body as far as you can, keeping your abdominals contracted to prevent yourself from jackknifing. Straighten your arms and push up without locking your elbows. Repeat as many times as you can.

    If you find this too difficult, do a modified push-up in which your knees are on the floor. If you find push-ups too easy, you can prop your feet on an exercise ball or an exercise block so that your body declines in relation to the floor.

2. *Squats.* Squatting develops balance and stability. It extends your back, increases mobility in your hips, lengthens your calves, stretches your Achilles tendons, and strengthens your knees and your ankles.

    With your knees and your feet together, your chest lifted, and your back straight, squat down as far as you can without losing your balance. Do not go any deeper than where you can control knee motion and do not let your back bend. Hold for a few seconds, stand up, and repeat.

    If you find this difficult or impossible, try squatting while holding on to the legs of a table or the back of a sturdy chair. You can also hold on to an elastic band tied to a doorknob. If you still can't do squats, squat into a chair or even a chair with pillows. Over time you'll evolve into doing a full squat.

As you practice the squat, the goal is to do more repetitions and squat deeper. If you are lifting weights and are strong enough, squatting with weights is an excellent exercise.

3. *Crunches.* Crunches develop abdominal strength and also strengthen your lower back.

   Lie on your back with your hands crossed on your chest or with your fingers touching the sides of your head (keep your elbows out to the side, not pointing up toward the ceiling). Place your feet on the floor with your legs bent. To begin the exercise, raise your torso, lifting your shoulder blades off the floor and crunching your rib cage toward your lower belly. Hold for two counts, then lower slowly to the starting position. Repeat.

   This is the basic crunch. There are dozens of variations with increasing levels of difficultly. If you are strong enough, you can do crunches at the gym on an inclined bench while holding weight plates on your chest. There are also machines at most gyms that mimic the motion of a crunch, and they can be set at various degrees of difficulty. We also like doing crunches while sitting on an exercise ball.

4. *Biceps curls.* Biceps curls are very adaptable. You can do them with barbells, dumbbells, or bands. You can even do them with any suitably heavy object, such as a soup can or a rock. Also, there are weight machines that duplicate this motion while keeping your arms from swinging, which would shift some of the stress from your biceps to your shoulders and chest (not good).

   Hold weights with your palms facing out, your elbows next to your body. Bend your elbows and curl the weights toward your shoulders without moving your elbows. Lower and repeat.

5. *Triceps dips.* It is very important to exercise both the biceps and the triceps to maintain balance in the strength of your arms.

Using a bench or a chair, sit with your hands next to or slightly under your hips. Lift up onto your hands and bring your hips forward. Bend the elbows (no less than ninety degrees) and lower your hips—keep them very close to the chair or bench. Don't scrunch up your shoulders. Push back up without locking your elbows, and repeat.

Most gyms have a dip machine with handles for doing triceps dips, and many gyms have a weight-counterbalanced dip machine that will let you do dips with various degrees of effort, from really easy to very hard.

6. *Static lunges.* Lunges are great for working all of the major muscles of the hips, glutes, and thighs.

   Stand up straight with your right foot forward and your left foot back about three feet. Hold a dumbbell in each hand, if desired, and bend your knees to lower your body toward the floor. Keep the knee behind your toes and be sure to lower straight down, not forward. Keep your torso straight and your stomach in tight as you push through the heel and back to a starting position. Repeat.

   As with the other exercises here, there are many variations, including front and reverse lunges and sliding lunges. By using increasingly heavy dumbbells, you can make lunges a permanent part of your routine even when you get to be stronger than Arnold Schwarzenegger.

7. *Grip squeezes.* Strengthening your grip, which is often overlooked by other exercise programs, is crucial for anyone who wants to live a long, healthy life. One of the key measures of muscle mass, grip strength has been correlated with longer life span in several studies and with lower blood pressure in others. We like it because we never want to be so weak that we can't open the lids of jars and bottles.

   If you don't have a hand gripper or if your gym doesn't have a grip trainer, you can do this simple grip-strengthening exercise with a washcloth or a hand towel. Thoroughly soak the cloth or towel with water, form it into a ball, and wring out the water as much as you can with one hand. Repeat with the other hand. Keep doing the grip exercises until your hands feel very tired and you can see that the veins in your hands and your wrists have expanded from the extra blood flow.

The Immortality Edge Fitness Forever Plan

Once you've developed your very own resistance routine, you can incorporate it into your Immortality Edge exercise program. You've finished the Six Weeks to Fitness plan and are ready to move on to the next phase, which we call the Fitness Forever Plan. You can either stay on the same level (one to four) or, if you feel ready, move on to a higher level. Once you're at level four, the goal is to increase not the amount of exercise but rather the intensity.

There are three distinct types of exercise in the Fitness Forever Plan: interval, endurance, and resistance. You can vary the program by changing the days and the number of times you do each type, as long as you do at least two days of interval training and one each of endurance and resistance. You can also do up to three days of each. The only rule is that you can't do resistance training two days in a row, because your muscles need an extra day to recover from this type of exercise. Remember, the goal is to increase the intensity of your efforts, not the amount of time you spend exercising. Once you feel ready, move up to the next level.

This plan is designed to keep you going for many years. So get going!

Level One

MONDAY

    5- to 10-minute stretching routine

    5-minute cardio warm-up

    30-second burst at 90% effort, increasing to 100% the final 10 seconds

90 seconds at a very slow pace without stopping

30-second burst at 90% effort, increasing to 100% the final 10 seconds

90 seconds at a very slow pace without stopping

End with a few more stretches

Total time: 19 minutes

TUESDAY

5- to 10-minute stretching routine

Resistance training: Do 3 sets of each exercise in your routine, 8–12 repetitions for each

Total time: 30 minutes

WEDNESDAY

Take a break but get some extra exercise by walking a bit more than usual or climbing some stairs you wouldn't otherwise climb.

THURSDAY

5- to 10-minute stretching routine

5-minute cardio warm-up

30-second burst at 90% effort, increasing to 100% the final 10 seconds

90 seconds at a very slow pace without stopping

30-second burst at 90% effort, increasing to 100% the final 10 seconds

90 seconds at a very slow pace without stopping

End with a few more stretches

Total time: 19 minutes

FRIDAY

5- to 10-minute stretching routine

Resistance training: Do 3 sets of each exercise in your routine, 8–12 repetitions for each

Total time: 30 minutes

SATURDAY

5- to 10-minute stretching routine

20 minutes cardio, with a 90% burst the last 30 seconds

Total time: 30 minutes

SUNDAY

Take a long leisurely walk, jog, or bike ride and enjoy being outdoors. If it is hot, go early in the morning. If it is cold, bundle up! Spend a few moments thinking about how good you feel, having completed your first week in phase two of the Immortality Edge exercise program, and how you are looking forward to next week.

Level Two

MONDAY

5- to 10-minute stretching routine

5-minute cardio warm-up

30-second burst at 90% effort, increasing to 100% the final 10 seconds

90 seconds at a very slow pace without stopping

30-second burst at 100% effort

90 seconds at a very slow pace without stopping

30-second burst at 100% effort

90 seconds at a very slow pace without stopping

30-second burst at 100% effort

90 seconds at a very slow pace without stopping

End with a few more stretches

Total time: 23 minutes

TUESDAY

5- to 10-minute stretching routine

Resistance training: Do 3 sets of each exercise in your routine, 8–12 repetitions for each.

Total time: 30 minutes

WEDNESDAY

Take a break but get some extra exercise by walking a bit more than usual or climbing some stairs you wouldn't otherwise climb.

THURSDAY

5- to 10-minute stretching routine

5-minute cardio warm-up

30-second burst at 90% effort, increasing to 100% the final 10 seconds

90 seconds at a very slow pace without stopping

30-second burst at 100% effort

90 seconds at a very slow pace without stopping

30-second burst at 100% effort

90 seconds at a very slow pace without stopping

30-second burst at 100% effort

90 seconds at a very slow pace without stopping

End with a few more stretches

Total time: 23 minutes

FRIDAY

5- to 10-minute stretching routine

Resistance training: Do 3 sets of each exercise in your routine, 8–12 repetitions for each.

Total time: 30 minutes

SATURDAY

5- to 10-minute stretching routine

25 minutes cardio, with a 90% burst the last 30 seconds

Total time: 35 minutes

SUNDAY

Take a long leisurely walk, jog, or bike ride and enjoy being outdoors. If it is hot, go early in the morning. If it is cold, bundle up! Spend a few moments thinking about how good you feel, having completed another week of the Immortality Edge exercise program, and how you are looking forward to next week.

Level Three

MONDAY

5- to 10-minute stretching routine
5-minute cardio warm-up
30-second burst at 90% effort
90 seconds at a very slow pace without stopping
30-second burst at 100% effort
90 seconds at a very slow pace without stopping
30-second burst at 100% effort
90 seconds at a very slow pace without stopping
30-second burst at 100% effort
90 seconds at a very slow pace without stopping
30-second burst at 100% effort
90 seconds at a very slow pace without stopping
30-second burst at 100% effort
90 seconds at a very slow pace without stopping
30-second burst at 100% effort
90 seconds at a very slow pace without stopping
End with a few more stretches

Total time: 29 minutes

TUESDAY

5- to 10-minute stretching routine
Resistance training: Do 5 sets of each exercise in your routine, 8–12 repetitions for each.

Total time: 45 minutes

WEDNESDAY

Take a break but get some extra exercise by walking a bit more than usual or climbing some stairs you wouldn't otherwise climb.

THURSDAY

5- to 10-minute stretching routine
5-minute cardio warm-up
30-second burst at 90% effort
90 seconds at a very slow pace without stopping
30-second burst at 100% effort
90 seconds at a very slow pace without stopping
30-second burst at 100% effort
90 seconds at a very slow pace without stopping
30-second burst at 100% effort
90 seconds at a very slow pace without stopping
30-second burst at 100% effort
90 seconds at a very slow pace without stopping
30-second burst at 100% effort
90 seconds at a very slow pace without stopping
30-second burst at 100% effort
90 seconds at a very slow pace without stopping
End with a few more stretches

Total time: 29 minutes

FRIDAY

5- to 10-minute stretching routine
Resistance training: Do 5 sets of each exercise in your routine,
    8–12 repetitions for each.

Total time: 45 minutes

SATURDAY

5- to 10-minute stretching routine
30 minutes cardio, with a 90% burst the last 30 seconds

Total time: 40 minutes

SUNDAY

Take a long leisurely walk, jog, or bike ride and enjoy being
    outdoors. If it is hot, go early in the morning. If it is cold,
    bundle up! Spend a few moments thinking about how good

you feel, having completed another week of the Immortality Edge exercise program, and how you are looking forward to next week.

Level Four

MONDAY

5- to 10-minute stretching routine

5-minute cardio warm-up

30-second burst at 90% effort, accelerating to 100% the last 10 seconds

90 seconds at a moderate pace without stopping

30-second burst at 90% effort, accelerating to 100% the last 10 seconds

90 seconds at a moderate pace without stopping

30-second burst at 100% effort

30-second pause

30-second burst at 100% effort

30-second pause

30-second burst at 100% effort

30-second pause

30-second burst at 100% effort

30-second pause

30-second burst at 100% effort

30-second pause

30-second burst at 100% effort

30-second pause

End with a few more stretches

Total time: 25 minutes

TUESDAY

5- to 10-minute stretching routine

Resistance training: Do 5 sets of each exercise in your routine, 8–12 repetitions for each.

Total time: 45 minutes

WEDNESDAY

Take a break but get some extra exercise by walking a bit more than usual or climbing some stairs you wouldn't otherwise climb.

THURSDAY

5- to 10-minute stretching routine

5-minute cardio warm-up

30-second burst at 90% effort, accelerating to 100% the last 10 seconds

90 seconds at a moderate pace without stopping

30-second burst at 90% effort, accelerating to 100% the last 10 seconds

90 seconds at a moderate pace without stopping

30-second burst at 100% effort

30-second pause

30-second burst at 100% effort

30-second pause

30-second burst at 100% effort

30-second pause

30-second burst at 100% effort

30-second pause

30-second burst at 100% effort

30-second pause

30-second burst at 100% effort

30-second pause

End with a few more stretches

Total time: 25 minutes

FRIDAY

5- to 10-minute stretching routine

Resistance training: Do 5 sets of each exercise in your routine, 8–12 repetitions for each.

Total time: 45 minutes

SATURDAY

5- to 10-minute stretching routine
45 minutes cardio, with a 100% burst the last 30 seconds

Total time: 55 minutes

SUNDAY

Take a long leisurely walk, jog, or bike ride and enjoy being outdoors. If it is hot, go early in the morning. If it is cold, bundle up! Spend a few moments thinking about how good you feel, having completed another week of the Immortality Edge exercise program, and how you are looking forward to next week.

GLOSSARY

active isolated stretching (AIS)   A form of stretching in which one muscle at a time is isolated, stretched, and strengthened.

adipokine   A chemical signal that comes from fat, usually pro-inflammatory in nature.

amyloid   A tangled web of protein substances that are usually broken down from healthy tissues or are leftovers from an inflammatory interaction within a tissue. These substances can be markers of damage or actually damaging in and of themselves, especially in the brain and the heart, where they can disrupt normal function.

antioxidant   A compound (often naturally occurring in fruits and vegetables or plants and herbs) that soaks up free radicals and decreases oxidation and inflammation in the body.

apoptosis   A genetically determined process of cell self-destruction in which a cell basically commits suicide. In many cases, the length of the telomere signals the time of apoptosis.

autophagy   A process in which the cells of the body are "eaten" and recycled to make use of valuable resources. It is a way of removing sick, dying, or dead cells from the body without wasting the useful components of those cells. As a person ages, the autophagocytic process is thought to become crippled and inefficient.

beta-sitosterol   One of several sterol (not to be confused with *steroid*) compounds found in certain nuts and vegetables that can directly lower cholesterol by interfering with its production or metabolism. Avocados and artichokes contain this compound.

biological age   The functional age of a cell and of a person. It is how young a cell behaves and performs in terms of its biochemical pathways and its telomere length. In a person, it is one's appearance, energy, and vitality, as measured by lab tests and tests of function such as lung and heart capacity.

body mass index (BMI)   A calculation of the amount of space the body occupies in square meters to generate a number that is compared to the rest of the population. A BMI of 25 is considered overweight and a BMI of 30 is considered obese. While the risk factors of being overweight and obese are similar, there is an approximate increase of 25 percent of those risk factors such as diabetes, arthritis, and vascular disease in obesity versus overweight. As one climbs up the BMI into the morbidly obese, generally considered a BMI of 40 or above, the risks get higher.

cardio   Exercise that stimulates the heart rate to go above its normal resting level. Effective cardio usually occurs at around 70 percent of the maximum heart rate.

carotenoid   A pigmented (yellow and orange) naturally occurring chemical from vegetables of the same colors, which contain certain nutrients.

cell replication   The division of one cell into two, which requires a complete copy of the DNA. Cell replication is part of the normal repair and growth process of a cell. Replication is done in such a way that the cell loses bits and pieces of DNA each time the cell divides. This DNA normally comes from the telomere and not the important gene material. Since the telomere determines the life span of the cell, each division shortens both the telomere and the life span of the cell.

chronological age   The actual age of a person in calendar years.

cognitive skill   The mind's ability to think and to process information.

c-reactive protein (CRP)   An inflammatory marker that can be measured through a simple blood test. It is considered a risk factor for vascular disease and blood vessel clogging.

DNA   The abbreviation for deoxyribonucleic acid, DNA is found in the chromosomes of all living cells. It is a coiled structure that contains most of the important genetic material. There are approximately 125,000 unique genes in the human genome, most of which are found on the chromosomes.

end products of glycation   The result of too much sugar attaching to various molecules in the body, which causes premature aging of the cells as well as disease.

EPA and DHA   The two essential fatty acid components of fish oil, eicosapentaenoic acid and docosahexaenoic acid. Conversion from a compound called alpha-linolenic acid (found in flaxseed) is possible in the body on a small scale. However, this does not happen with enough efficiency to meet the levels that are required to offset the high level of inflammatory fatty acids present in today's typical American diet.

fast-twitch muscle fiber   A muscle fiber that is capable of storing sugar or oxygen for fuel and is responsible for strength, endurance, or repetitive efforts of fairly high but not maximal intensity. It is somewhere between slow twitch and ultra-fast twitch.

flash point   The point at which cooking oil starts to burn.

flavonoid   A colored compound in vegetables, roots, and flowers that creates antioxidant actions in the body. It can help to rid the body of chemicals or compounds that cause mutations of the DNA and cancer.

free radical   A highly unstable nitrogen or oxygen molecule that is capable of oxidizing and damaging cells and cellular material. Free radicals are normally contained in the mitochondria as a by-product of fuel generation and are used when necessary to create an inflammatory response or cause the cell to undergo apoptosis. Free radicals can be good or bad, depending on their amounts or the situations in which they are present. Based on our current understanding of disease and health, most people have far too many free radicals.

frontal cortex and prefrontal cortex   The areas of the brain where higher intellectual functions and decision-making processes reside. These areas are activated in meditative states.

gene   One of a complete packet of inherited material that codes for a specific characteristic; for example, eye color. Genes are made up of sequences of DNA and are grouped together to form chromosomes. A human being has forty-six chromosomes in the nucleus of each cell and a circular chromosome in the mitochondria.

genetic expression   The quality of being "read" or made into something. Not all genes are expressed. Some may exist in the genome and never produce anything; these are called *repressed* or *unexpressed*.

glutathione   A very simple molecule that is a combination of three amino acids: cysteine, glycine, and glutamine. It is often called the "master of all antioxidants" because it plays a major role in preventing aging, cancer, heart disease, dementia, and more, and it is necessary to treat everything from autism to Alzheimer's disease. The body produces its own glutathione, but it can be depleted by poor diet, pollution, toxins, medications, stress, trauma, aging, infections, and radiation.

glycation The attachment of sugar molecules to other vital molecules or chemical compounds inside or outside the cell that impairs their functions and causes damage.

glycemic index (G-I) The rate at which a food raises blood sugar, compared to either table sugar (sucrose) or intravenous glucose (depending on which scale is used). Sucrose has a G-I of 85, and intravenous glucose has a G-I of 100. Below 55 is acceptable as a low-glycemic food.

glycogen Stored sugar in the muscles and the liver that is available for short high-intensity exercise or for endurance exercise; it lasts less than three hours. Once it is exhausted, a condition occurs in the muscles referred to as *glycogen depletion* or, more commonly, "the wall."

Hayflick limit The theoretical number of times that any cell can divide, which indicates its potential life span. The Hayflick limit for normal human (somatic) cells is about 120 years. The Hayflick limit is named after Leonard Hayflick, the microbiologist who discovered in 1962 that cultured normal human and animal cells have a limited capacity for replication.

homocysteine An amino acid (a protein building block) that is part of a critical antioxidant cycle that occurs naturally in the human body. Homocysteine elevation is often due to deficiencies in B_6 or other B vitamins and can be a serious source of inflammation in the body as well as an independent risk factor for stroke and heart disease.

human growth hormone (HGH) A hormone released by the pituitary gland that causes the liver to release another hormone that circulates throughout the body, causing increased fat metabolism and muscle growth. It is also active in many other tissues, including the brain, the heart, and other glands or endocrine organs, influencing their function.

immune surveillance The role of the immune system in policing the body to get rid of cancer cells.

inflammation A process in which the immune system creates an environment that oxidizes, or burns, certain cells or tissues in the body. Normally part of the defense system against bacteria and viruses as well as of normal repair and tissue turnover, it can become the root of many of the disease processes of aging if it is not controlled and properly regulated.

interval training Short repeated bursts of high-intensity effort geared to increasing the heart rate above 86 percent of its maximum and keeping it there for a short time, resulting in breathlessness, followed by complete or nearly complete recovery.

maximum heart rate   The fastest rate at which the heart can safely beat. The formula for an approximate calculation is 220 minus your age. Thus, if you are fifty years old, your maximum heart rate is approximately 170 beats per minute. Athletes in training can often safely exceed this level.

mean telomere length (MTL)   The standard laboratory method of reporting white blood cell telomere length, consisting of an average value for a large sample of white blood cell telomeres.

methylation   One of many on-off switches in the body thought to control bad genes and promote good genes. Lack of methylation in the telomeres is associated with shorter than normal telomeres in several diseases, including Parkinson's.

mitochondria   The powerhouses of the cell that burn fat and oxygen to make fuel. Mitochondria also contain short circular chromosomes that house the rest of the important genetic material in the cell. Mitochondria are part of the loop that tells the cell it is "time to die." This process, apoptosis, is a kind of explosion from within the cell and is triggered by short telomeres or severely damaged DNA.

mutation   A change in the DNA of a gene that leads to something different from what was originally present in the genetic material; it is often bad and is thought to be the result of oxidation and inflammation.

N-acetylcysteine (NAC)   A potent antioxidant amino acid and sulfur donor. It was originally used, and is still used today, for acetaminophen overdoses.

neurotransmitter   A substance that carries a chemical message from one nerve to another, causing a response.

nutraceutical   A food, herb, or dietary supplement that has druglike actions in the body and can influence the outcomes of diseases.

nutrigenomics   The study of how food and supplements affect the human genetic code.

omega-3 fatty acids   A "good" fat found largely in fish that promotes heart, circulatory, and brain health. Omega-3 has been shown to prevent premature telomere shortening and oxidation. It also helps to control genetic expression.

omega-6 fatty acids   Pro-inflammatory essential fatty acids that are necessary in the diet but are present in our current diet in far too large amounts, leading to generalized inflammation in the body. This in turn may lead to premature telomere shortening. Omega-6 also controls genetic expression.

oncogene(s)   A gene that promotes or causes cancer.

oxidation   The process of combining oxygen molecules known as free radicals to destroy certain tissues and initiate the inflammatory response.

oxidative stress   A functional measure of how much oxidation is in the body. Because no direct single direct measurement exists, oxidative stress is indirectly measured by several substitute measurements. These include the ratio of omega-6 to omega 3, C-reactive protein (CRP), homocysteine levels, interleukin-6, and others. The tests for these are available from your doctor, but some of them are not routinely done or covered by insurance.

oxygen debt   A condition that occurs when primarily fast-twitch fibers are used for an activity. The energy they burn up in sugar creates by-products that require increased oxygen and more rapid breathing to restore the body to its usual operating range. It is indicated by increased breathing or heavy panting, if the exercise is intense enough.

phytonutrient   A compound that occurs naturally in fruits and vegetables; it has both foodlike and vitaminlike qualities. An example would be lycopene from tomatoes and watermelon.

polychlorinated biphenyls (PCBs)   A class of widely used organic compounds that do not break down rapidly in the environment and have become pollutants. Toxicities vary, but their persistence in the food chain, particularly in water-based foods such as fish and shellfish, has made them commonly ingested pollutants in people. PCBs are linked to cancer, birth defects, rashes, and numerous other reactions.

polyphenols   A class of pigmented antioxidants that come from berries, green tea, and other natural sources.

resistance training   Training with muscular force against any kind of resistance, including weights, kettle bells, weight machines, bands, and even your own body weight.

senescence   The state in which a cell stops replicating and slowly winds down toward death. Senescent cells are sick and dying and place an abnormal load on the rest of the tissues and the body if there are a lot of them.

short telomere   A telomere with five thousand or fewer base pairs. It is approaching the end of its clock function and is responsible for signaling to the cell that it is "time to die." Short telomeres are usually the only ones that matter, in terms of longevity.

slow-twitch muscle fiber   The type of fiber that makes up the bulk of the muscle fibers in the body. It is good for endurance.

smoke point   The point at which a cooking fat starts to smoke, which signifies the start of significant oxidation of that oil. Foods that are cooked in oil should be cooked in oils with high smoke points.

sprint 8   An interval-training program, developed by Phil Campbell, that consists of eight intervals of thirty-second maximal exertions followed by ninety seconds of slow speed.

stem cell   A precursor cell that can become any other kind of cell and is kept in reserve so the body can generate new cells of different types when they are needed. Telomerase is more active in these cells than in somatic (body) cells but is less active than in reproductive cells.

stress chemical: cortisol   A steroid hormone that temporarily decreases inflammation but that over time leads to immune suppression bone loss and fat storage, resulting in an inflammatory state.

stress chemicals: epinephrine and norepinephrine   Short-acting fight-or-flight chemicals whose increase leads to dilated eyes, rapid heart rate, high blood pressure, and tremors.

sympathetic and parasympathetic nervous systems   Nerve systems that control the flow and level of activation of many of the endocrine glands and organs, including the heart, the lungs, and the intestines. Considered to be automatic and to generate automatic response in most people, these nervous systems are intimately linked to the effects of stress, anxiety, and meditation.

TA-65   The only known and tested telomerase activator to be successfully used in humans. It is derived from a single molecule that is a rare component of the astragalus plant. Attempts to copy TA-65's structure and function have not met with success, so TA-65 remains the only telomerase activator with positive proof of effect that is in commercial use by people all over the world.

telomerase   An enzyme that makes telomeres longer and gives cells immortality. Only some cells (reproduction cells and cancer cells) have it turned on in high enough amounts to be potentially immortal. Stem cells have lower telomerase activity than reproduction cells but higher telomerase activity than the cells in the rest of the body. The latter have no or little telomerase, because the gene is covered up or repressed, which prevents telomerase from being made.

telomerase activator A chemical that removes the repression for most cells and allows telomerase to be expressed, thus lengthening the cells' telomeres.

telomere A short repetitive segment of nongenetic material that functions as a biological clock to determine the life span of a cell (that is, how many times it can reproduce before it dies). The telomere is also intimately involved with stabilizing the genetic material and is thus directly involved in the health of the cell and the entire organism.

transcendental meditation (TM) A unique form of mantra meditation that requires a structured course and a certified teacher. Originated by Maharishi Mahesh Yogi and popularized by the Beatles, it is practiced all over the world by hundreds of thousands of people for its mental and physical benefits.

tumor suppressor gene A gene that inhibits or prevents the growth of cancer.

ultra-fast-twitch muscle fiber A fiber that is responsible for intense explosive movements of very short duration.

ultraviolet (UV) light Solar radiation from sunlight and some forms of artificial light that consists of A rays and B rays, both of which can cause oxidation and inflammation if the exposure is too high.

yoga An Indian traditional practice that combines postures, breathing, meditation, and stretching to achieve an enlightened state of total mental and bodily flexibility.

RESOURCES

Apps for Smart Phones and Tablet Computers (Fitness, Health, Nutrition, and Meditation)

Android

http://101bestandroidapps.com

http://androidapps.com

Apple

http://appcraver.com

http://appsforipad.net

http://apple.com/iphone/apps-for-everything/working-out.html

http://appsafari.com

http://appstoreapps.com/most-popular-apps/

Online Resources

Fitness

Body Mass Index Calculator

http://exrx.net/Calculators/BMI.html

Cyberdiet

www.cyberdiet.com

Equinox Fitness Centers

www.equinox.com

Exercise TV

http://exercisetv.tv

Fitness.com

http://fitness.com

Firstpath

http://firstpath.com

Fitness Online

http://fitnessonline.com

Greta Blackburn's Fit Camp
   http://fitcamp.com
Gym America
   http://gymamerica.com
Health and Fitness at Web MD
   www.webmd.com/fitness-exercise
Institute of Human Performance
   http://ihpfit.com
Internet Fitness
   www.internetfitness.com
Map My Run
   www.mapmyrun.com
Men's Fitness
   www.mensfitness.com
My Fitness Page
   www.myfitnesspage.com/
Phil Campbell's High-Intensity Sprinting
   www.bodybuilding.com/fun/phil3.htm
Women's Fitness
   www.womenfitness.net
Yoga Today
   www.yogatoday.com

Holistic Medical Information
Arizona Center for Integrative Medicine
   http://integrativemedicine.arizona.edu
Capella Online University: What's Next in Health
   www.whatsnextnetwork.com/health
Healthline
   www.healthline.com
Holistic Health Yellow Pages
   www.findhealer.com
Medical News Today
   www.medicalnewstoday.com
Dr. Joseph Mercola
   http://mercola.com
Microsoft Health Vault
   www.healthvault.com
Natural Eye Care
   www.naturaleyecare.com

Natural News
www.naturalnews.com
Natural Solutions for Health
www.healthy.net
Third Age
www.thirdage.com
Women's Health
www.ivillage.com
Dr. Dave Woynarowski
http://drdavesbest.com

Life Extension Organizations
Alcor Life Extension Foundation
www.alcor.org
American Academy of Anti-Aging Medicine
www.worldhealth.net
American Federation for Aging Research
www.afar.org
BioTime, Inc.
www.biotimeinc.com
Geron Corporation
www.geron.com
Life Extension Foundation
http://lef.org
Longevity Meme
www.longevitymeme.org
Manhattan Beach Project to Cure Aging by 2029
http://manhattanbeachproject.com
Maximum Life Foundation
http://maxlife.org
National Institute on Aging
www.nia.nih.gov
Repeat Diagnostics
http://repeatdiagnostics.com
SENS (Strategies for Engineered Negligible Senescence) Foundation
www.sens.org
Sierra Sciences
http://sierrasciences.com
Spectracell Laboratories
http:/spectracell.com

Stanford Center on Longevity
http://longevity.stanford.edu
T. A. Sciences
http://tasciences.com
Telonauts
http://telonauts.com

Meditation

How to Meditate
www.how-to-meditate.org
Learning Meditation
www.learningmeditation.com
Meditation Videos
http://youtube.com
Enter "meditation" in the search box.
Realization
http://realization.org
Transcendental Meditation
www.tm.org
Wildmind Buddhist Meditation
http://wildmind.org
World Wide Meditation Center
www.meditationcenter.com

Nutrition

About Nutrition
http://nutrition.about.com
All Recipes
http://allrecipes.com
Calorie Counter
http://newcaloriecounter.com
Cooking Light
www.cookinglight.com
Diabetic Living
www.diabeticlivingonline.com
Diet Facts
http://dietfacts.com
Diet Journal and Calorie Counter
www.my-calorie-counter.com
Food Fit
http://foodfit.com

Glycemic Index
   www.glycemicedge.com
   www.glycemicindex.com
Nutrition Data
   www.nutritiondata.com
Nutrition Navigator from Tufts University
   http://navigator.tufts.edu
Nutrition Portal
   www.thenutritionportal.com
World's Healthiest Foods
   www.whfoods.com
Zuvo Pure Water
   http://zuvowater.com

Supplements
Dr. Dave's Best
   www.drdavesbest.com
Life Extension Foundation
   www.lef.org
Nutraceuticals World
   www.nutraceuticalsworld.com
Signals Stem Cell Solution Cream
   www.signals120.com
Supplement Watch
   www.supplementwatch.com
Vita Search
   www.vitasearch.com

Yoga
Baron Baptiste Vinyasa Yoga
   www.baronbaptiste.com
Suza Francina Yoga
   www.suzafrancina.com
Bryan Kest Power Yoga
   www.poweryoga.com
Stephanie Culen Sacred Strength Yoga
   www.stephanieculen.com

REFERENCES

Introduction: The Hunt for Immortality

Atzmon, G., M. Cho, R. M. Cawthon, et al. "Evolution in Health and Medicine Sackler Colloquium: Genetic Variation in Human Telomerase Is Associated with Telomere Length in Ashkenazi Centenarians." *Proceedings of the National Academy of Sciences* (January 26, 2010): Suppl. 1:1710–1717.

Brady, Catherine. *Elizabeth Blackburn and the Story of Telomeres: Deciphering the Ends of DNA.* Cambridge, MA: MIT Press, 2007.

Chiang, Y. J., R. T. Calado, K. S. Hathcock, et al. "Telomere Length Is Inherited with Resetting of the Telomere Set-Point." *Proceedings of the National Academy of Sciences* (May 17, 2010). www.pnas.org/content/early/2010/05/07/0913125107.abstract.

De Grey, A., N. Bostrom, and A. Sandberg. *Why Should We Live Forever?* New Scientist Video, October 10, 2007. www.youtube.com/watch?v=XfTqXL0d9Ls.

Dreifus, Claudia. "A Conversation with Carol W. Greider." *New York Times*, October 12, 2009.

Fakhoury J., D. T. Marie-Egyptienne, J. A. Londono-Vallejo, et al. "Telomeric Function of Mammalian Telomerases at Short Telomeres." *Journal of Cell Science* 123, no. 10 (May 15, 2010): 1693–1704.

Fossel, Michael. *Reversing Human Aging.* New York: William Morrow, 1996.

Huber, Peter. "The FDA and Methuselah." *Forbes*, April 12, 2010.

Kipling, D., T. Davis, E. L. Ostler, and G. A. Faragher. "What Can Progeroid Syndromes Tell Us about Human Aging?" *Science* 305 (5689) (2004): 1426–1431.

Maximum Life Foundation. *BioTime Reverses the Age of Human Cells!* March 16, 2010. http://maxlifefoundation.com.

Rodriguez-Brenes, I. A., and C. S. Peskin. "Quantitative Theory of Telomere Length Regulation and Cellular Senescence." *Proceedings of the National Academy of Sciences of the United States of America* 107, no. 12 (March 23, 2010): 5387–5392.

Sierra Sciences. *Bill Andrews on Telomere Basics: Curing Aging.* www .sierrasciences.com/telomere.

U.S. Census Bureau. "World Population Summary." International Date Base. www.census.gov/ipc/www/idb/worldpopinfo.php.

Watson, James D. *The Double Helix: A Personal Account of the Discovery of the Structure of DNA.* London: Weidenfeld and Nicholson, 1997.

1. The Aging Cure

Andrews, William. "Telomerase Activation: The Future of Anti-Aging Medicine." Presentation at the American Academy of Anti-Aging Conference, September 11, 2009. www.youtube.com/watch?v=F3breSdC UXA&feature=related.

Cooney, C. A. "Are Somatic Cells Inherently Deficient in Methylation Metabolism? A Proposed Mechanism for DNA Methylation Loss, Senescence and Aging." *Growth, Development and Aging* 57, no. 4 (Winter 1993): 261–273.

De Grey, Aubrey, and Michael Rae. *Ending Aging: The Rejuvenation Breakthroughs That Could Reverse Human Aging in Our Lifetime.* New York: St. Martin's Press, 2007.

Freitas, Robert A., Jr. *Nanomedicine: Basic Capabilities.* Vol. 1. Austin, TX: Landes Bioscience, 1999.

Grossman, Terry, and Ray Kurzweil. *Fantastic Voyage: Live Long Enough to Live Forever.* New York: Rodale Press, 2004.

Gugliucci, A. "Glycation as the Glucose Link to Diabetic Complications." *Journal of the American Osteopathic Association* 100, no. 10 (2000): 621–634.

Gugliucci, A., K. Mehlhaff, E. Kinugasa, et al. "Paraoxonase-1 Concentrations in End-Stage Renal Disease Patients Increase after Hemodialysis: Correlation with Low Molecular AGE Adduct Clearance." *International Journal of Clinical Chemistry* 377 (2007): 213–220.

Kendrick, Mandy. "Anti-Aging Pill Targets Telomeres at the Ends of Chromosomes." *Scientific American*, August 2009.

Marquez, F. Z., M. A. Markus, and B. J. Morris. "The Molecular Basis of Longevity, and Clinical Implications." *Maturitas* 65, no. 2 (February 2010): 87–91.

Mount Sinai Medical Center. "Study Shows That Reducing Processed and Fried Food Intake Lowers Related Health Risks and Restores Body's

Defenses." Press release (November 4, 2009). www.mountsinai.org/
about-us/newsroom/press-releases/study-shows-that-reducing-proc-
essed-and-fried-food-intake-lowers-related-health-risks-and-restores-
bodys-defenses.

Olshansky, S. J., Perry, D., Miller, R. A., et al. "In Pursuit of the Longevity Dividend: What Should We Be Doing to Prepare for the Unprec-
edented Aging of Humanity?" *The Scientist* (March, 2006).

Simm, A., J. Wagner, T. Gursinsky, et al. "Advanced Glycation Endprod-
ucts: A Biomarker for Age as an Outcome Predictor after Cardiac Surgery?" *Experimental Gerontology* 42, no. 7 (July 2007): 668–675.

2. The Immortality Edge Supplement Plan

Ames, B. N., H. Atamna, and D. W. Killilea. "Mineral and Vitamin
Deficiencies Can Accelerate the Mitochondrial Decay of Aging."
Molecular Aspect of Medicine 25, no. 4–5 (August–October 2005):
363–378.

Andron, L., N. A. Gavan, I. A. Veresiu, et al. "In Vivo Effect of Lipoic Acid
on Lipid Peroxidation in Patients with Diabetic Neuropathy." *In Vivo*
14, no. 2 (March 2000): 327–330.

Armas, L. A. G., B. W. Hollis, and R. Heaney. "Vitamin D_2 Much Less
Effective Than Vitamin D_3 in Humans." *Journal of Clinical Endocrinology
and Metabolism* (2004): 5387–5391.

Borras, C., J. M. Esteve, J. R. Vina, et al. "Glutathione Regulates Telomerase Activity in 3T3 Fibroblasts." *Journal of Biological Chemistry* 89,
no. 11 (August 2004): 34332–34335.

Bruning, Nancy, and Shari Lieberman. *The Real Vitamin and Mineral Book*.
Knoxville, TN: Avery, 2007.

Calabrese, V., C. Cornelius, A. T. Dinkova-Kostova, et al. "Vitagenes,
Cellular Stress Response, and Acetylcarnitine: Relevance to Hormesis."
Biofactors 35, no. 2 (March–April 2009): 146–160.

Choi, J., S. R. Fauce, and R. B. Effros. "Reduced Telomerase Activity
in Human T Lymphocytes Exposed to Cortisol." *Brain, Behavior, and
Immunity* 22, no. 4 (May 2008): 600–605.

Engelhart, M. J., M. I. Geerlings, A. Ruitenberg, et al. "Diet and Risk of
Dementia: Does Fat Matter? The Rotterdam Study." *Neurology* 59, no.
12 (2003): 2020–2021.

Farzaneh-Far, R., J. Lin, E. S. Epel, et al. "Association of Marine Omega-
3 Fatty Acid Levels with Telomeric Aging in Patients with Coronary
Heart Disease." *Journal of the American Medical Association* 33, no. 3
(January 20, 2010): 250–257.

Gleissman, H., J. I. Johnsen, and P. Kogner. "Omega-3 Fatty Acids in Cancer: The Protectors of Good and the Killers of Evil?" *Experimental Cell Research* 316, no. 8 (May 2010): 1365–1373.

Khalsa, Soram. *The Vitamin D Revolution: How the Power of This Amazing Vitamin Can Change Your Life*. London: Hay House, 2009.

Kilham, Chris. "The Healing Powers of Elderberry." Medicine Hunter. http://medicinehunter.com/elderberry2.htm.

Kirby, David. *Animal Factory: The Looming Threat of Industrial Pig, Dairy, and Poultry Farms to Humans and the Environment*. New York: St. Martin's Press, 2010.

Moneysmith, Marie. *Basic Health Publications User's Guide to Carnosine*. Laguna Beach, CA: Basic Health, 2004.

Natural Products Insider. "Major Fish Oil Products Face Prop 65 Suit." March 2, 2010. www.naturalproductsinsider.com.

Richards, J. B., A. M. Valdes, J. P. Gardner, et al. "Higher Serum Vitamin D Concentrations Are Associated with Longer Leukocyte Telomere Length in Women." *American Journal of Clinical Nutrition* 86, no. 5 (November 2007): 1420–1425.

Richter, T., and T. von Zglinkicki. "A Continuous Correlation between Oxidative Stress and Telomere Shortening in Fibroblasts." *Experimental Gerontology* 42, no. 11 (November 2007): 1039–1042.

Rodriquez-Hernandez, A., M. D. Cordero, L. Salviati, et al. "Coenzyme Q Deficiency Triggers Mitochondria Degradation by Mitophagy." *Autophagy* 5, no. 1 (January 2009): 19–32.

Roschek, B., Jr., R. C. Fink, M. D. McMichael, et al. "Elderberry Flavonoids Bind to and Prevent H1N1 Infection in Vitro." *Phytochemistry* 70, no. 10 (July 2009): 1255–1261.

Saretzki, G., M. P. Murphy, and T. von Zglinkicki. "MitoQ Counteracts Telomere Shortening and Elongates Lifespan of Fibroblasts under Mild Oxidative Stress." *Aging Cell* 2, no. 2 (April 2003): 141–143.

Shao L., Q. H. Li, and Z. Tan. "L-Carnosine Reduces Telomere Damage and Shortening Rate in Cultured Normal Fibroblasts." *Biochemical and Biophysical Research Communications* 324, no. 2 (November 2004): 931–936.

Sinatra, Stephen P. *The Coenzyme Q_{10} Phenomenon*. New York: McGraw-Hill, 1998.

T. A. Sciences. "About TA-65." www.tasciences.com.

Wang, L., J. E. Manson, Y. Song, et al. "Systematic Review: Vitamin D and Calcium Supplementation in Prevention of Cardiovascular Events." *Annals of Internal Medicine* 152, no. 5 (March 2010): 315–323.

Xu, Q., C. G. Parks, L. A. DeRoo, et al. "Multivitamin Use and Telomere Length in Women." *American Journal of Clinical Nutrition* 89, no. 6 (June 2009): 1857–1863.

3. The Immortality Edge Fitness Plan

Barbieri, M., G. Paolisso, M. Kimura, et al. "Higher Circulating Levels of IGF-1 Are Associated with Longer Leukocyte Telomere Length in Healthy Subjects." *Mechanisms of Aging and Development* 130, no. 11–12 (November–December 2009): 771–776.

Campbell, Phil. *Ready, Set, Go! Synergy Fitness for Time-Crunched Adults.* Jackson, TN: Pristine, 2008.

Cherkas, L. F., J. L. Hunkin, B. S. Kato, et al. "The Association between Physical Activity in Leisure Time and Leukocyte Telomere Length." *Archives of Internal Medicine* 168, no. 2 (January 28, 2008): 154–158.

Gibala, M. "Molecular Responses to High-Intensity Interval Exercise." *Applied Physiology, Nutrition and Metabolism* 34, no. 3 (June 2009): 428–432.

Godfrey, R. J. "The Exercise-Induced Growth Hormone Response in Athletes." *Sports Medicine* 33, no. 8 (2003): 599–613.

Grant, S., K. Corbett, K. Todd, et al. "A Comparison of Physiological Responses and Rating of Perceived Exertion in Two Modes of Aerobic Exercise in Men and Women over 50 Years of Age." *British Journal of Sports Medicine* 36, no. 4 (February 2002): 276–281.

Larson, E., L. Wang, J. D. Bowen, et al. "Exercise Is Associated with Reduced Risk for Incident Dementia among Persons 65 Years of Age and Older." *Annals of Internal Medicine* 144, no. 2 (January 17, 2006): 73–81.

Mora, S., R. F. Redberg, Y. Cui, et al. "Ability of Exercise Testing to Predict Cardiovascular and All-Cause Death in Asymptomatic Women." *Journal of the American Medical Association* 290, no. 12 (September 24, 2003): 1600–1607.

Rae, D. E., A. Vignaud, G. S. Butler-Browne, et al. "Skeletal Muscle Telomere Length in Healthy, Experienced, Endurance Runners." *European Journal of Applied Physiology* 109, no. 2 (May 2010): 323–330.

Rantanen, T., J. M. Guralnik, D. Foley, et al. "Midlife Hand Grip Strength as a Predictor of Old Age Disability." *Journal of the American Medical Association* 281, no. 6 (1999): 558–560.

Richardson, C. R., A. M. Kriska, P. M. Lantz, et al. "Physical Activity and Mortality across Cardiovascular Disease Risk Groups." *Medicine and Science in Sports and Exercise* 36, no. 11 (November 2004): 1923–1929.

Scott, C. B. "Contributions of Anerobic Energy Expenditure to Whole Body Thermogenesis." *Nutrition and Metabolism* 48, no. 4 (June 2005): 14.

4. The Immortality Edge Stress-Reduction Plan

Blackburn, Elizabeth. "Stress, Telomeres and Telomerase in Humans." University of California–San Francisco, Department of Biochemistry and Biophysics. http://ibioseminars.org/blackburn/blackburn3.shtml.

Creswell, J. D., B. M. Way, N. I. Eisenberger, and M. D. Lieberman. "Neural Correlates of Dispositional Mindfulness during Affect Labeling." *Psychosomatic Medicine* 69, no. 6 (July–August 2004): 560–565.

Dear, J. W., K. Gough, and D. J. Webb. "Transcendental Meditation and Hypertension." *Postgraduate Medical Journal* 84, no. 994 (August 2008): 417.

Dreifus, Claudia. "Finding Clues to Aging in the Fraying Tips of Chromosomes: A Conversation with Elizabeth H. Blackburn." *New York Times*, July 3, 2007.

Epel, E. S., E. H. Blackburn, J. Lin, et al. "Accelerated Telomere Shortening in Response to Life Stress." *Proceedings of the National Academy of Sciences of the United States of America* (September 28, 2004). www.pnas.org/content/101/49/17312.

Epel, E. S., J. Daubenmier, J. T. Moskowitz, S. Folkman, and E. Blackburn. "Can Meditation Slow Rate of Cellular Aging? Cognitive Stress, Mindfulness, and Telomeres." *Annals of New York Academy of Sciences* 1172 (August 2009): 34–53.

Epel, E. S., J. Lin, F. S. Dhabber, et al. "Dynamics of Telomerase Activity in Response to Acute Psychological Stress." *Brain, Behavior and Immunity* 24, no. 4 (May 2010): 531–539.

Lutz, A., H. A. Slagter, N. B. Rawlings, et al. "Mental Training Enhances Attentional Stability: Neural and Behavioral Evidence." *Journal of Neuroscience* 29, no. 42 (October 2009): 13417–13427.

Siegel, Ronald. *The Mindfulness Solution: Everyday Practices for Everyday Problems.* New York: Guilford Press, 2009.

U.S. Department of Health and Human Services, National Institutes of Health. "NIH-Funded Scientific Research on Transcendental Meditation." www.tmeducation.org/research-national-institutes-of-health.

Valdes, A. M., I. J. Deary, J. Gardner, et al. "Leukocyte Telomere Length Is Associated with Cognitive Performance in Healthy Women." *Neurobiology of Aging* 31, no. 6 (June 2010): 986–992.

Zeidan, F., S. K. Johnson, B. J. Diamond, et al. "Mindfulness Meditation Improves Cognition: Evidence of a Brief Mental Training." *Consciousness and Cognition* 19, no. 2 (June 2010): 597–605.

5. Add Years to Your Life

Babizhayev, M. A., E. L. Savel'yeva, S. N. Moskvina, et al. "Telomere Length Is a Biomarker of Cumulative Oxidative Stress, Biologic Age, and an Independent Predictor of Survival and Therapeutic Treatment Requirements Associated with Smoking Behavor." *American Journal of Therapeutics* (March 29, 2010). http://journals.lww.com/americanthera peutics/Abstract/publishahead/Telomere_Length_is_a_Biomarker_of_ Cumulative.99779.aspx.

Bakaysa, S. L., L. A. Mucci, P. E. Slagboom, et al. "Telomere Length Predicts Survival Independent of Genetic Influences." *Aging Cell* 6, no. 6 (October 6, 2007): 709–713.

Bunnell, David, and Frederic J. Vagnini. *Count Down Your Age.* New York: McGraw-Hill, 2007.

Fossel, Michael. *Cells, Aging, and Human Disease.* New York: Oxford University Press, 2004.

Jones, Megan. "50 Online Tests and Tools to Calculate Your Health and Wellness." www.nursingschoolsearch.com/blog/2008/07/50-online-tests-and-tools-to-calculate-your-health-wellness.

Kurzweil, Ray, and Terry Grossman. *Fantastic Voyage: The Science behind Radical Life Extension.* New York: Penguin, 2004.

Loayza, D., and T. de Lange. "Telomerase Regulation at the Telomere: A Binary Switch." *Cell* 117, no. 3 (April 30, 2004): 279–280.

RealAge. "Are You Younger or Older Than Your Calendar Age? Take the RealAge Test and Find Out." www.realage.com.

SpectraCell Laboratories. www.spectracell.com.

6. The Immortality Edge Forever Nutrition Plan

Alderman, M. "Reducing Dietary Sodium: The Case for Caution." *Journal of the American Medical Association* 303, no. 5 (2010): 448–449.

Berquin, I. M., Y. Min, R. Wu, et al. "Modulation of Prostate Cancer Genetic Risk by Omega-3 and Omega-6 Fatty Acids." *Journal of Clinical Investigation* 117, no. 7 (2007): 1866–1875.

Brand-Miller, J., J. McMillan-Price, K. Steinbeck, et al. "Carbohydrates—the Good, the Bad and the Whole Grain." *Asia Pacific Journal of Clinical Nutrition* 17, Suppl. 1 (2008): 16–19.

Carlsen, M. H., B. L. Halvorsen, K. Holte, et al. "The Total Antioxidant Content of More Than 3100 Foods, Beverages, Spices, Herbs and Supplements Used Worldwide." *Nutrition Journal* 9, no. 3 (January 22, 2010). www.nutritionj.com/content/9/1/3.

Cassidy, A., I. D. Vivo, Y. Liu, et al. "Associations between Diet, Lifestyle Factors, and Telomere Length in Women." *American Journal of Clinical Nutrition* 91, no. 5 (May 2010): 1273–1278.

Chan, R., J. Woo, E. Suen, et al. "Chinese Tea Consumption Is Associated with Longer Telomere Length in Elderly Chinese Men." *British Journal of Nutrition* 103, no. 1 (January 2010): 107–113.

Chao, A., M. J. Thun, C. J. Connell, et al. "Meat Consumption and Risk of Colorectal Cancer." *Journal of the American Medical Association* 293, no. 2 (2005): 172–182.

Cordain, Loren. *The Paleo Diet.* New York: John Wiley & Sons, 2002.

Farzaneh-Far, R., J. Lin, E. S. Epel, et al. "Association of Marine Omega-3 Fatty Acid Levels with Telomeric Aging in Patients with Coronary Heart Disease." *Journal of the American Medical Association* 303, no. 3 (2010): 250–257.

Fraser, G. E., and D. J. Shavik. "Ten Years of Life: Is It a Matter of Choice?" *Archives of Internal Medicine* 1, no. 13 (July 9, 2001): 1645–1652.

Harvard School of Public Health. "Results from Large, Long Women's Health Initiative Dietary Modification Trial Show No Effect on Heart Disease, Breast Cancer, Colorectal Cancer, or Weight." May 28, 2010. www.hsph.harvard.edu/.

Johnson, Nathan. "Swine of the Times: The Making of the Modern Pig." *Harper's*, May 2006.

Kiefer, A., J. Lin, E. Blackburn, et al. "Dietary Restraint and Telomere Length in Pre- and Postmenopausal Women." *Psychosomatic Medicine* 70, no. 8 (October 2008): 845–849.

Konstantinova, S. V., G. S. Tell, S. E. Vollset, et al. "Dietary Patterns, Food Groups, and Nutrients as Predictors of Plasma Choline and Betaine in Middle-Aged and Elderly Men and Women." *American Journal of Clinical Nutrition* 88, no. 6 (2008): 1663–1669.

National Academy of Sciences, Institute of Medicine, Food and Nutrition Board. "Dietary Reference Intakes: Recommended Intakes for Individuals." October 23, 2009. http://fnic.nal.usda.gov/nal_display/index.php?info_center=4&tax_level=2&tax_subject=256&topic_id=1342.

Natural Resources Defense Council. "Safety Matters When Selecting Fish and Sushi." January 2008. www.simplesteps.org/food/shopping-wise/safety-matters-when-selecting-fish-and-sushi.

Nestle, Marion. *What to Eat*. New York: North Point Press, 2006.

O'Callaghan, N. J., P. M. Clifton, M. Noakes, et al. "Weight Loss in Obese Men Is Associated with Increased Telomere Length and Decreased Abasic Sites in Rectal Mucosa." *Rejuvenation Research* 12, no. 3 (June 2009): 169–176.

Ocampo, C. "Telomere Talk: The Nutrition Connection." *Journal of Nutrition for the Elderly* 29, no. 1 (January 2010): 110–111.

Raloff, Janet. "Reevaluating Eggs' Cholesterol Risk." *Science News*, June 2006.

Scudder, B. C., L. C. Chaser, D. A. Wentz, et al. *Mercury in Fish, Bed Sediment, and Water from Streams across the United States* (2009). United States Geological Survey, U.S. Department of the Interior. http://pubs .usgs.gov/sir/2009/5109/pdf/sir20095109.pdf.

Song, W. O., and J. M. Kerver. "National Contribution of Eggs to American Diets." *Journal of the American College of Nutrition*. October 19 (5 Suppl.) (2000): 556–562.

Willett, Walter C. *Eat, Drink, and Be Healthy*. New York: Free Press, 2001.

INDEX

CPSIA information can be obtained at www.ICGtesting.com
Printed in the USA
LVOW06s0205050116

469060LV00001B/329/P